The Everyday Survival Pantry

How to Prepare for the Unthinkable

Personal Use Permission

Readers are welcome to print copies of this book for their own personal use or for use within their household. This permission does not allow the reproduction, resale, redistribution, or commercial use of this book in any form. No part of this publication may be copied, reproduced, or distributed for sale, shared publicly online, or republished in any format without written permission from the author.

This book is intended for informational and educational purposes only. While every effort has been made to ensure the accuracy of the information contained in this publication, the author makes no guarantees regarding the completeness or suitability of the information provided. The author assumes no responsibility for any loss, injury, or damage resulting from the use of the information contained in this book. Food preparation, storage, and safety practices may vary depending on local conditions. Readers are encouraged to follow appropriate food safety guidelines and exercise their own judgment.

First Edition

Author: Michele Withonel

ISBN: 978-1-7645345-3-6

Contents

Introduction

Having a well-stocked pantry is one of the simplest and most practical ways to support food security for you and your household. Non-perishable foods are items that can be safely stored at room temperature for extended periods without spoiling, making them an essential part of everyday meal planning and emergency preparedness.

These foods are especially useful for:

- Emergency preparedness
- Busy households
- Budget-friendly meal planning
- Reducing frequent grocery trips
- Long-term food storage

Non-perishable foods include canned, dried, freeze-dried, and packaged products that can remain safe and nutritious for months or even years when stored correctly. Because of their long shelf life, they provide a reliable foundation for meals when fresh foods are not available or when shopping becomes difficult.

This book is designed as a practical guide to building and maintaining a well-organised pantry while showing how simple shelf-stable ingredients can be used to prepare nourishing and satisfying meals. Within these pages, you will find **approximately 240 recipes made primarily from pantry**

ingredients, demonstrating how everyday shelf-stable foods can be transformed into a wide variety of breakfasts, lunches, breads, pastries, dinners, desserts, sauces, and quick meals.

Recognising that many households also care for pets, this book also includes **13 simple recipes for pet food and treats** that can be prepared using pantry ingredients when regular pet supplies may be limited. In addition, there are **11 recipes for basic cleaning and hygiene solutions**, using common household items that can help maintain cleanliness and sanitation when commercial products are unavailable.

To support practical preparation, this guide also includes several useful checklists designed to help readers build a well-prepared household. These include:

- A comprehensive non-perishable pantry food checklist
- A non-food emergency supply checklist
- A prepared household checklist to help organise essential supplies

These tools are designed to help readers gradually build a reliable pantry and household supply system that supports both everyday living and unexpected situations.

Non-perishable foods are often referred to as **shelf-stable foods**, meaning they can be stored safely at room temperature without refrigeration or freezing before they are opened. Unlike fresh foods such as meat, dairy, or produce, these foods are processed or packaged in ways that slow the growth of bacteria and microorganisms that cause spoilage.

Because of this, shelf-stable foods are particularly valuable in situations such as:

- Power outages
- Natural disasters
- Remote travel or camping
- Budget-conscious grocery planning
- Busy households needing quick meal options

When selected thoughtfully, non-perishable foods can provide essential nutrients, including protein, carbohydrates, fats, vitamins, and minerals. By combining a variety of these foods, it is possible to create balanced meals that support both nutrition and practicality.

This book aims to show that with a little planning and a well-stocked pantry, households can prepare simple, nourishing meals, maintain basic household needs, and feel more confident when facing everyday challenges or unexpected disruptions.

Building a Well-Stocked Pantry

A thoughtfully stocked pantry is an important part of maintaining a well-organised and resilient household. Non-perishable foods are convenient and long-lasting, but a well-planned pantry should also include a variety of foods that support balanced nutrition while providing flexibility for everyday cooking and unexpected situations.

A balanced pantry typically includes foods from several key categories:

- **Protein sources** such as canned fish, beans, lentils, or nut butters.
- **Grains and carbohydrates** such as rice, pasta, oats, and cereals.
- **Fruits and vegetables** in canned, dried, or freeze-dried form.
- **Dairy or dairy alternatives** such as powdered milk or shelf-stable milk.
- **Fats and oils** are used for cooking, flavour, and energy.

By combining foods from these groups, it is possible to prepare nutritious and satisfying meals using only shelf-stable ingredients. Many simple pantry meals can be created by pairing grains with protein sources and adding vegetables, sauces, or seasonings for flavour and variety.

Maintaining a supply of non-perishable foods offers several practical benefits for households of all sizes. Pantry staples provide convenience for everyday cooking while also helping families prepare for situations when fresh food may not be readily available.

One of the most important reasons to keep a pantry stocked is **emergency preparedness**. Unexpected situations such as severe weather, natural disasters, transportation disruptions, illness, power outages or war can temporarily limit access to grocery stores. During these times, having shelf-stable foods available ensures that households can still prepare safe and nutritious meals. Because many pantry foods require little preparation and do not need refrigeration before opening, they remain usable for an extended time.

A well-stocked pantry also provides **convenience** in daily life. Busy schedules, work commitments, and family responsibilities can sometimes make frequent grocery shopping difficult. With staple ingredients already available at home, meals can often be prepared quickly and easily. Pantry foods such as rice, pasta, canned vegetables, and beans can be combined with sauces, herbs, or spices to create a wide range of simple and satisfying dishes.

Another benefit of maintaining a pantry is the potential for **cost savings**. Shelf-stable foods can often be purchased in bulk or during sales, reducing the cost per item. Staples such as rice, pasta, oats, dried beans, and canned goods store well for long periods and can help households build an affordable and dependable food supply. Because these foods last longer than many fresh items, they are also less likely to spoil before being used, which helps reduce food waste.

Perhaps most importantly, maintaining a pantry can provide **peace of mind**. Knowing that your household has a reliable supply of food available can reduce stress and provide reassurance during uncertain situations. Even a modest pantry stocked with essential items can help ensure that meals remain possible when shopping trips are delayed or unexpected events occur.

Building a non-perishable pantry does not need to happen all at once. Many households gradually add shelf-stable foods during regular grocery trips. Over time, this approach creates a dependable food supply that supports both everyday cooking and emergency preparedness.

With thoughtful planning and regular use, a well-balanced pantry can become one of the most valuable and practical resources when the unexpected happens.

Why Non-Perishable Foods Last

Food preservation methods are used to extend the shelf life of foods by reducing moisture, limiting oxygen exposure, or sealing foods in protective containers. These processes help prevent the growth of bacteria, yeast, and mould. Some of the most common preservation methods include:

Canning

Canning involves sealing food in airtight containers and heating them to destroy harmful microorganisms. The heating process creates a vacuum seal that prevents bacteria from entering the container.

Common canned foods include:

- Vegetables such as corn, peas, and beans.
- Fruits such as peaches and pineapple.
- Meats and fish such as tuna, salmon, and chicken.
- Soups and ready-to-eat meals.

Properly canned foods can last **several years when stored correctly**.

Dehydration

Dehydration removes moisture from food through controlled drying. Since microorganisms require moisture to grow, removing water significantly slows spoilage.

Examples of dehydrated foods include:

- Dried fruits such as raisins and apricots.
- Dried vegetables.
- Jerky and dried meats.
- Powdered milk and powdered eggs.

Dehydrated foods are lightweight, compact, and easy to store, making them popular for long-term storage and outdoor activities.

Freeze-Drying

Freeze-drying is an advanced preservation method that removes moisture by freezing food and then slowly extracting the ice as vapour. This process preserves much of the food's original texture, flavour, and nutritional value.

Common freeze-dried foods include:

- Fruits such as strawberries and blueberries.
- Vegetables such as peas and corn.
- Meats and prepared meals.

Freeze-dried foods are often used for **long-term emergency food storage** because they can last many years when sealed properly.

Vacuum Sealing

Vacuum sealing removes air from packaging before sealing it. Since oxygen contributes to food spoilage and oxidation, removing it helps extend shelf life.

Vacuum sealing is commonly used for:

- Dried foods.
- Coffee and tea.
- Nuts and seeds.
- Long-term grain storage.

This method is often combined with other preservation techniques to further extend storage life.

Airtight Packaging

Many packaged foods are sealed in airtight containers or packaging materials that protect the food from moisture, oxygen, and contaminants.

Examples include:

- Pasta and noodles.
- Rice and grains.
- Crackers and cereals.
- Snack foods and baking ingredients.

Proper packaging helps ensure the food remains fresh until opened.

Shelf Life and Proper Storage

Although non-perishable foods last much longer than fresh foods, proper storage conditions are still important for maintaining their quality, flavour, and safety. Storing foods correctly can significantly extend their shelf life and help prevent spoilage.

To maximise shelf life, foods should be stored in an environment that is:

- **Cool** – ideally below normal room temperature when possible.
- **Dry** – moisture can lead to mould, spoilage, or damaged packaging.
- **Dark** – light can reduce quality and degrade some foods, particularly oils and dried products.

Pantries, cupboards, and cool storage areas are often ideal locations for storing shelf-stable foods. Avoid areas that experience **high humidity, direct sunlight, or extreme heat**, as these conditions can shorten the shelf life of many foods.

It is also important to ensure that food packaging remains intact. If original packaging becomes damaged or opened, transfer the contents to **clean, airtight containers** to protect the food from moisture, pests, and contamination. Labelling containers with the **purchase or storage date** can also help you keep track of how long foods have been stored.

From time to time, check stored foods for:

- Damaged or compromised packaging
- Expired or approaching best-before dates
- Signs of spoilage such as swollen cans, rust, leaks, or unusual odours

A helpful way to maintain a well-organised pantry is to rotate foods regularly using the **First-In, First-Out (FIFO)** method. This simply means using older items first and replacing them with newer purchases. Rotating food supplies helps keep your pantry fresh, reduces waste, and ensures that foods are used while they are still at their best quality.

With proper storage and regular rotation, a well-stocked pantry can provide reliable and long-lasting food supplies for everyday meals as well as unexpected situations.

Stocking a Resilient Pantry

A thoughtfully stocked pantry makes meal preparation easier and reduces the need for frequent grocery trips. When basic ingredients are always available, simple meals can be prepared quickly using a combination of pantry staples and fresh foods.

A practical pantry usually includes foods from several major food groups such as grains, proteins, fruits and vegetables, and healthy fats. Keeping a range of ingredients on hand helps ensure that meals remain both satisfying and nutritionally balanced.

It is also helpful to include a mix of ingredients that can be used in cooking as well as items that require little or no preparation. This combination allows households to prepare full meals when time permits while still having convenient options available during busy days or unexpected situations.

The following steps provide a simple approach to building a pantry that is organised, balanced, and easy to maintain.

Protein Sources

Protein is an essential nutrient that plays a vital role in maintaining overall health. It helps build and repair body tissues, supports muscle strength, and contributes to many important functions within the body. Proteins are made up of amino acids, which are often referred to as the building blocks of life because they are used to create and maintain cells, enzymes, and hormones.

Including adequate protein in the diet is important for people of all ages. Protein helps support muscle development, assists in repairing tissues after injury or physical activity, and plays a key role in maintaining a strong immune system. It also helps the body feel satisfied after meals, which can contribute to sustained energy levels throughout the day.

In addition to supporting muscle health, protein contributes to several other important bodily functions, including:

- Supporting healthy skin, hair, and nails.
- Helping produce enzymes and hormones.
- Assisting in the transport of nutrients throughout the body.
- Supporting immune system function.

For these reasons, it is important that meals include a reliable source of protein.

Fortunately, many shelf-stable foods provide excellent protein options that can be stored in a pantry for long periods. These foods are particularly valuable because they remain safe to consume without refrigeration until opened, making them ideal for everyday cooking as well as emergency food storage.

Common non-perishable protein sources include:

• Canned meats and fish such as tuna, salmon, and chicken.
• Canned beans and legumes such as black beans, chickpeas, and lentils.
• Dried beans and lentils that can be stored for extended periods.
• Nut butters such as peanut butter and almond butter.
• Powdered protein products such as powdered eggs or protein powder.

These foods can easily be incorporated into a wide variety of meals. For example, canned beans can be added to soups and rice dishes, tuna can be used in salads or pasta, and nut butters can be paired with crackers or oats for quick and nutritious snacks.

Combining protein foods with grains and vegetables can help create balanced meals that provide both energy and essential nutrients. Keeping a variety of shelf-stable protein sources in your pantry ensures that you always have the ingredients needed to prepare filling and nutritious meals.

Canned Meats and Fish

Canned protein sources are convenient and ready to eat.

Examples include:

- Tuna.
- Salmon.
- Chicken.
- Turkey.
- Sardines.
- Corned beef.

These are often packed in water, oil, or sauces to extend shelf life.

They can be used in:

- Sandwiches.
- Salads.
- Pasta dishes.
- Rice meals.
- Casseroles.

Dried and Freeze-Dried Meats

These options are lightweight and have a very long shelf life.

Examples include:

- Beef jerky.
- Turkey jerky.
- Beef sticks.
- Freeze-dried chicken.

These foods are excellent for:

- Snacks.
- Travel.
- Emergency food kits.
- Backpacking.

Canned Beans and Legumes

Beans and legumes are excellent plant-based protein sources.

Common varieties include:

- Black beans.
- Kidney beans.
- Chickpeas.
- Lentils.
- Split peas.

Dried beans can last up to **10 years or longer** when stored properly.

They are perfect for:

- Soups.
- Stews.
- Salads.
- Rice dishes.

Nut Butters

Nut butters are nutritious, filling, and long-lasting.

Examples include:

- Peanut butter.
- Almond butter.
- Cashew butter.

These spreads contain:

- Protein.
- Healthy fats.
- Vitamins and minerals.

They can be eaten with crackers, bread, fruit, or added to smoothies and sauces.

Powdered Protein Sources

Powdered proteins are useful for cooking or adding nutrition to meals.

Examples include:

- Protein powders.
- Powdered eggs.
- Soy protein powder.

These can be used in:

- Baking.
- Smoothies.
- Pancakes.
- Emergency meal replacements.

Grains and Carbohydrates

Carbohydrates provide the body with energy and play an important role in maintaining balanced and satisfying meals. They are the body's primary source of fuel and help support everyday activities such as working, exercising, and maintaining normal bodily functions.

When consumed, carbohydrates are broken down into glucose, which the body uses to produce energy for the brain, muscles, and other organs. Because of this, carbohydrate-rich foods are an essential part of a healthy and balanced diet.

Many common pantry staples are excellent sources of carbohydrates. Foods such as rice, pasta, oats, cereals, and flour-based products are widely used in households around the world and can be stored for long periods when kept in proper conditions.

In addition to providing energy, many carbohydrate foods also supply important nutrients such as:

- Dietary fibre, which supports digestive health.
- B vitamins, which help the body convert food into energy.
- Essential minerals such as iron and magnesium.

Whole grains, in particular, are valued for their nutritional benefits because they provide fibre and additional nutrients that contribute to overall health. Carbohydrate foods are also extremely versatile in meal preparation. They serve as the foundation for many dishes and can be combined with proteins, vegetables, and sauces to create filling and balanced meals.

For example:

- Rice can be paired with beans, canned vegetables, or meats.
- Pasta can be served with tomato sauce, tuna, or vegetables.
- Oats can be prepared as a warm breakfast or used in baking.
- Flour and baking mixes can be used to make breads, pancakes, and other baked goods.

Because many grain-based foods are dried or packaged, they are ideal for long-term pantry storage. When stored in airtight containers in a cool, dry location, many carbohydrate foods can remain fresh for months or even years.

Including a variety of grains and other carbohydrate-rich foods in your pantry helps ensure that you always have a reliable source of energy and a flexible base for preparing nutritious meals.

Rice

Rice is one of the most common pantry staples. Types include:

- White rice.
- Brown rice.
- Jasmine rice.
- Basmati rice.

White rice generally has the **longest shelf life**.

Rice pairs well with:

- Beans.
- Canned vegetables.
- Meat.
- Sauces.

Pasta and Noodles

Dried pasta stores easily and cooks quickly. Examples include:

- Spaghetti.
- Macaroni.
- Penne.
- Ramen noodles.

Pasta is versatile and can be combined with canned sauces, vegetables, and proteins.

Oats and Cereals

Whole grains provide fibre and long-lasting energy.

Examples include:

- Rolled oats.
- Instant oats.
- Granola.
- Whole-grain cereals.

Oats are especially useful because they can be used in:

- Breakfast meals.
- Baking.
- Energy bars.

Flour and Baking Mixes

Baking staples allow you to prepare breads, pancakes, and other foods. Common options include:

- All-purpose flour.
- Whole wheat flour.
- Cornmeal.
- Pancake mix.

These ingredients expand the variety of meals you can prepare using pantry items.

Vegetables

Vegetables are an important part of a balanced diet and provide essential vitamins, minerals, fibre, and antioxidants that help support overall health. They contribute to digestion, immune function, and general well-being while also adding colour, flavour, and texture to meals.

Although fresh vegetables are commonly used in cooking, many vegetables are also available in **shelf-stable forms**, making them ideal for pantry cooking and emergency food supplies. Canned, dried, and freeze-dried vegetables retain many of their nutrients and can be stored for long periods without refrigeration.

Common pantry vegetables include canned corn, peas, green beans, carrots, mushrooms, potatoes, tomatoes, and mixed vegetables. Dried vegetables such as onion flakes, garlic, and dehydrated vegetable mixes are also useful for adding flavour to soups, stews, casseroles, and rice dishes.

Keeping a variety of shelf-stable vegetables in the pantry allows you to easily add nutrition, colour, and flavour to meals. They can be used in many different recipes, including soups, curries, pasta dishes, casseroles, and savoury pastries. By combining vegetables with grains, legumes, and protein sources, it is possible to create well-balanced meals even when fresh ingredients are not available.

Canned Vegetables

Canned vegetables are affordable and easy to store. Examples include:

- Corn.
- Peas.
- Green beans.
- Carrots.
- Tomatoes.
- Mixed vegetables.

They are useful for soups, stews, casseroles, and side dishes.

Dehydrated or Freeze-Dried Vegetables

These vegetables retain nutrients and store well for long periods. They are often used in soups, rice dishes, and pasta sauces. Examples include:

- Spinach.
- Kale.
- Bell peppers.
- Mushrooms.

Shelf-Stable Vegetable Sauces

Sauces add flavour and variety to meals.

Examples include:

- Tomato paste.
- Salsa.
- Vegetable-based pasta sauces.

These products help turn simple pantry ingredients into flavourful meals.

Fruits

Fruits are a valuable part of a balanced diet and provide natural sweetness along with important vitamins, minerals, fibre, and antioxidants. Many fruits are rich in vitamin C and other nutrients that support immune health, digestion, and overall well-being. They also add colour, flavour, and variety to meals and snacks.

While fresh fruits are widely enjoyed, many fruits are also available in **shelf-stable forms**, making them ideal for pantry cooking and long-term food storage. Canned fruits, dried fruits, and freeze-dried fruits can be stored for extended periods and still retain much of their nutritional value.

Common pantry fruits include canned peaches, pears, pineapple, apples, and fruit cocktail. Dried fruits such as raisins, apricots, cranberries, dates, and dried apples are also convenient and easy to store. Freeze-dried fruits are another option that provide long shelf life while preserving flavour and nutrients.

Shelf-stable fruits can be used in many ways in the kitchen. They can be added to breakfast cereals and oatmeal, baked into cakes and pastries, mixed into desserts, or used in savoury dishes such as curries, rice meals, and salads. They also make a convenient snack on their own.

Keeping a variety of fruits in your pantry helps ensure that meals remain both nutritious and enjoyable, providing natural sweetness and essential nutrients even when fresh produce is not available.

Canned Fruits

Popular canned fruits include:

- Peaches.
- Pineapple.
- Pears.
- Fruit cocktail.

They can be eaten as snacks or added to desserts and breakfasts.

Dried Fruits

Dried fruits are concentrated sources of nutrients. Examples include:

- Raisins.
- Apricots.
- Dates.
- Figs.
- Cranberries.

They are great for snacking or adding to cereals and baked goods.

Freeze-Dried Fruits

Freeze-dried fruits retain flavour and nutrients while lasting much longer.

Examples include:

- Strawberries.
- Blueberries.
- Apples.

They are lightweight and ideal for long-term storage.

Dairy and Dairy Alternatives

Dairy products and dairy alternatives are valuable sources of important nutrients, particularly **calcium, protein, and vitamins** that support strong bones, muscle health, and overall well-being. Including dairy or dairy alternatives in a pantry helps ensure that meals remain nutritionally balanced, even when fresh refrigerated foods are not available.

While many dairy products normally require refrigeration, several options are available in **shelf-stable forms** that can be safely stored for long periods. These products are especially useful for pantry cooking, baking, and emergency food supplies.

Common shelf-stable dairy products include **powdered milk, evaporated milk, sweetened condensed milk, powdered cheese, and shelf-stable long-life milk**. These ingredients can be used in a wide range of recipes, including baked goods, sauces, soups, desserts, and breakfast dishes such as oatmeal or cereal.

For those who prefer non-dairy options or have dietary restrictions, a variety of **plant-based alternatives** are also available in shelf-stable packaging. Examples include almond milk, soy milk, oat milk, rice milk, and coconut milk. These alternatives often provide similar versatility in cooking and baking while offering options for people who avoid traditional dairy products.

Shelf-stable dairy and dairy alternatives can be used in many everyday meals. They can be added to hot drinks such as coffee or tea, mixed into cereals and oatmeal, used in baking recipes, or incorporated into creamy sauces and soups. Products such as coconut milk are also commonly used in curries, desserts, and savoury dishes.

By keeping a selection of dairy or dairy alternatives in the pantry, households can easily add **flavour, texture, and nutritional value** to meals. These ingredients help support balanced nutrition while allowing a wide variety of recipes to be prepared using shelf-stable foods.

Powdered Milk

Powdered milk is commonly used in cooking and baking.

Dairy options include:

- Whole milk powder.
- Skim milk powder.

Non-dairy options include:

It can also be mixed with water for drinking.

- Soy milk powder.
- Coconut milk powder.
- Oat milk powder.
- Almond milk powder.

Evaporated and Sweetened Condensed Milk

These canned milk products are useful pantry staples with a long shelf life. They can be used in both cooking and baking.

Examples include:

- Evaporated milk.
- Sweetened condensed milk.

Non-Dairy Evaporated Milk Alternatives

Some plant-based products are made to mimic the thicker texture of evaporated milk. These may include:

- Evaporated coconut milk.
- Evaporated oat milk.
- Evaporated soy milk.

Non-Dairy Sweetened Condensed Milk Alternatives

Plant-based sweetened condensed milk is becoming more widely available. Examples include:

- Sweetened condensed coconut milk.
- Sweetened condensed oat milk.
- Sweetened condensed soy milk.

Shelf-Stable Plant-Based Milk

These milks are packaged to remain safe without refrigeration until opened. Examples include:

- Almond milk.
- Soy milk.
- Oat milk.
- Rice milk.

Powdered Cheese

Powdered cheese or cheese sauces add flavour to meals.

They can be used in:

- Pasta dishes
- Sauces.
- Soups.

Fats and Oils

Fats and oils play an important role in cooking and nutrition. They provide a concentrated source of energy and help add flavour, texture, and richness to many dishes. Fats are also necessary for the body to absorb certain vitamins, including vitamins A, D, E, and K.

In the kitchen, fats and oils are widely used for a variety of cooking methods such as frying, sautéing, roasting, and baking. They also help prevent foods from sticking to cooking surfaces and can improve the taste and texture of many recipes.

Many fats and oils are naturally **shelf-stable**, making them well suited for pantry storage. Common examples include vegetable oil, olive oil, coconut oil, and shortening. Other long-lasting options include ghee (clarified butter), nut butters such as peanut butter or almond butter, and seed-based products such as tahini.

These ingredients are extremely versatile and can be used in a wide range of dishes. Oils are commonly used when cooking grains, vegetables, and proteins.

Proper storage helps maintain the quality of fats and oils. They should generally be kept in a **cool, dark place**, as exposure to heat and light can cause oils to spoil more quickly. When stored correctly, many cooking oils can remain usable for extended periods.

Common pantry fats include:

- Vegetable oil.
- Olive oil.
- Coconut oil.
- Ghee.
- Shortening.
- Lard.

These ingredients are essential for frying, baking, and flavouring food.

Snacks and Convenience Foods

Snack foods and convenience items can be useful additions to a well-stocked pantry. They provide quick energy, add variety to meals, and offer simple options for times when preparing a full meal may not be practical.

Many snack foods are naturally shelf-stable and can be stored for extended periods without refrigeration. Examples include crackers, rice cakes, granola bars, protein bars, nuts, trail mix, dried fruit, pretzels, and packaged snack foods. These items can be enjoyed on their own or paired with other pantry ingredients such as nut butters, canned fish, or dried fruits to create more satisfying snacks.

Convenience foods can also be helpful when time is limited or when cooking facilities are not available. Ready-to-eat foods, instant noodles, instant soups, and packaged meal mixes can provide quick meal solutions using minimal preparation. These items are especially valuable during busy days, travel, camping trips, or emergency situations.

Snack foods can also play a role in maintaining energy levels throughout the day. Small snacks between meals can help provide sustained energy, particularly when they include a combination of carbohydrates, protein, and healthy fats.

While snacks are often enjoyed for convenience and enjoyment, they can also contribute to balanced eating when chosen thoughtfully. Including a variety of options in the pantry ensures that there are quick, accessible foods available for both everyday use and unexpected situations.

By keeping a selection of shelf-stable snacks and convenience foods on hand, households can add flexibility to their pantry while ensuring that quick and satisfying food options are always available. These items are helpful during busy days or emergencies.

Condiments, Spices, and Sweeteners

Condiments, spices, and sweeteners play an important role in the pantry by adding flavour, aroma, and variety to meals. While they may not always be the main ingredients in a dish, these flavouring items can transform simple pantry staples into more enjoyable and satisfying meals.

Many condiments and seasonings are naturally shelf-stable and can be stored for long periods when kept in a cool, dry place. Common examples include salt, pepper, dried herbs, spice blends, soy sauce, vinegar, mustard, hot sauce, and bouillon or broth powders. These ingredients help enhance the taste of foods such as rice, beans, pasta, vegetables, and soups.

Spices and herbs are especially valuable in pantry cooking because they allow the same basic ingredients to be prepared in different ways. For example, garlic powder, onion powder, paprika, cumin, curry powder, oregano, and chilli flakes can be used to create a wide range of flavours inspired by different cuisines.

Sweeteners are another important pantry item. Sugar, honey, maple syrup, and molasses can be used in baking, desserts, beverages, and even some savoury recipes. These ingredients help balance flavours and add sweetness to foods such as oatmeal, pastries, sauces, and marinades.

By keeping a variety of condiments, spices, and sweeteners in the pantry, it becomes much easier to prepare meals that are both flavourful and satisfying. Even simple combinations of grains, beans, or vegetables can be transformed into delicious dishes with the right seasonings.

A well-stocked collection of flavouring ingredients adds creativity and flexibility to pantry cooking, helping ensure that meals remain enjoyable even when using basic shelf-stable foods.

Sweeteners

• Sugar • Honey.• Syrup.

Honey can last **indefinitely** when stored properly.

Herbs and Spices

There are lots of Herbs and Spices but here are some examples:

- Oregano.
- Cummin.
- Cinnamon.
- Chilli powder.
- Garlic powder.

Spices transform simple foods into flavourful meals.

Shelf-Stable Sauces

Common options include:

- Soy sauce.
- Hot sauce.
- Ketchup.
- Mustard.
- Vinegar.

These sauces enhance the taste of many dishes.

Beverages

Shelf-stable beverages are an important part of a well-stocked pantry. They provide convenient drink options that can be stored for long periods and prepared whenever needed. Having a variety of beverages available helps ensure that households always have access to refreshing or comforting drinks, even when fresh supplies are limited.

Many beverages can be stored in pantry form, including coffee, tea, cocoa mixes, malted drink powders such as Milo or Ovaltine, and powdered drink mixes. These products typically have long shelf lives and require only water or milk to prepare. Instant coffee and tea are especially convenient because they can be made quickly with minimal equipment.

Powdered drink mixes and electrolyte beverages can also be useful additions to a pantry. These drinks can help provide hydration and flavour, particularly during hot weather, illness, or situations where plain water may become less appealing over time.

Shelf-stable milk and milk alternatives, such as long-life milk, almond milk, soy milk, oat milk, or powdered milk, can also be used in beverages and cooking. These products are helpful for preparing hot drinks like coffee, tea, and cocoa, as well as for use in cereals, baking, and other recipes.

Beverages also provide comfort and familiarity during stressful or unexpected situations. A warm cup of tea or coffee can offer a sense of routine and relaxation, while flavoured drinks can add variety to daily hydration.

By keeping a selection of shelf-stable beverages in the pantry, households can ensure they always have drink options available for everyday use as well as for emergencies.

Protecting Your Pantry from Pests

When storing non-perishable foods for extended periods, it is important to protect them from pests such as ants, mice, cockroaches, and pantry insects. These pests are attracted to food sources and can damage packaging or contaminate stored foods if proper precautions are not taken.

Taking a few simple steps can help keep your pantry clean, organised, and pest-free while ensuring that your stored foods remain safe and usable.

Store Foods in Airtight Containers

One of the most effective ways to protect pantry foods is to store dry goods in **airtight containers**. Foods such as flour, rice, pasta, oats, cereals, dried fruit, and nuts should be transferred into sealed containers made of glass, metal, or durable plastic.

Airtight containers help:

- Prevent insects and rodents from reaching the food
- Protect foods from moisture and humidity
- Keep foods fresher for longer

If the original packaging becomes damaged or opened, transferring the contents into sealed containers provides an additional layer of protection.

Keep the Pantry Clean

Regular cleaning helps prevent pests from becoming established. Wipe down shelves periodically and remove crumbs, spills, or open packaging that could attract insects or rodents. Good cleaning practices include:

• Wiping shelves regularly, • Sweeping or vacuuming pantry floors
• Removing empty packaging promptly, • Cleaning up spills immediately

Keeping the pantry clean reduces the food sources that attract pests.

Inspect Food Packages

Before storing newly purchased foods, check the packages for any signs of damage. Small holes, tears, or crushed boxes can allow insects or rodents to enter.

If packaging appears compromised, transfer the contents into sealed containers before storing the food.

Store Food Off the Floor

Whenever possible, store pantry items on shelves rather than directly on the floor. This helps improve air circulation and makes it easier to monitor for signs of pests.

Keeping food slightly elevated also makes cleaning easier and allows you to detect problems early.

Check Stored Foods Regularly

Periodically inspect pantry items for signs of pests or spoilage. Look for:

- Small holes or gnaw marks in packaging
- Insects inside containers or boxes
- Droppings or debris on shelves
- Unusual odours or damaged packaging

Early detection allows problems to be addressed before they spread.

Natural Deterrents

Some natural substances may help discourage pests in pantry areas. Bay leaves, cloves, or peppermint oil are sometimes used as mild deterrents for certain insects.

While these methods are not guaranteed to prevent pests, they may help reduce pest activity when combined with good storage practices.

Common Pantry Insects

Even well-maintained pantries may occasionally encounter insects that are attracted to stored foods. Some of the most common pantry pests include:

- **Weevils** – small beetles often found in grains, rice, and flour
- **Pantry moths** – moths whose larvae feed on cereals, grains, nuts, and dried foods
- **Flour beetles** – insects that infest flour, cereal, and grain products

These insects are often introduced into the home through packaged foods purchased from stores. Their eggs may already be present in dry foods such as grains or flour.

Preventing Pantry Insects

To reduce the risk of infestations:

- Store grains and flour in airtight containers
- Check packages before storing them
- Avoid keeping open food in its original packaging for long periods
- Rotate pantry foods regularly using the **first-in, first-out (FIFO)** method

Some people also freeze newly purchased grains or flour for a few days before storing them. Freezing can help destroy any insect eggs that may be present.

If an Infestation Occurs

If insects are discovered in pantry foods, it is best to discard the affected items and thoroughly clean the surrounding shelves and containers. Washing storage containers with warm, soapy water and drying them completely before refilling can help prevent further problems.

Maintaining a Healthy Pantry

A clean, organised pantry combined with proper storage practices greatly reduces the risk of pest problems. By storing foods in sealed containers, inspecting items regularly, and keeping storage areas clean, pantry foods can remain safe and fresh for long periods.

Protecting your pantry from pests helps ensure that your stored food supply remains reliable and ready to use for everyday meals as well as unexpected situations.

Recipes for Disasters and Other Unexpected Events.

The recipes in this section are designed to show how simple pantry ingredients can be transformed into satisfying, nourishing meals. Many people believe that cooking requires fresh ingredients, specialty products, or complicated techniques. In reality, some of the most practical and reliable meals can be made using foods that store well and are commonly found in the pantry.

These recipes focus on using **shelf-stable ingredients that are affordable, versatile, and easy to store**. With items such as grains, beans, canned foods, dried goods, and basic cooking staples, it is possible to prepare a wide range of meals without relying on fresh ingredients or frequent shopping trips.

This collection includes recipes for everyday cooking as well as situations when resources may be limited. You will find simple breakfasts, hearty lunches, breads and traditional damper, savoury pastries, quick dinners, and meals built around pantry staples such as beans, grains, and canned fish. There are also recipes for sauces, flour-based survival meals, no-cook dishes, and quick meals that can be prepared in under twenty minutes.

Because comfort and variety are also important, the section includes sweet recipes as well. You will find cakes, pastries, desserts, candies, and treats that can be made using ingredients that store well in the pantry. There are even a few familiar favourites for those days when the kids simply want something quick and comforting.

The goal of these recipes is not perfection, but practicality. They are designed to be **flexible, adaptable, and forgiving**, allowing you to use the ingredients you already have on hand. Many recipes can easily be adjusted depending on what is available in your pantry. Whether you are cooking an everyday meal, preparing food during a busy week, or relying on stored foods during an unexpected situation, these recipes demonstrate that **simple ingredients can still produce nourishing and satisfying meals**.

Breakfast

Breakfast doesn't require fresh ingredients to be nourishing and comforting. With a well-stocked pantry, you can create warm, satisfying breakfasts using oats, canned fruit, powdered milk, nut butters, grains, and simple baking staples.

These recipes are designed to be **easy, affordable, and made mostly from shelf-stable foods**—perfect for busy mornings, emergencies, camping trips, or simply making the most of your pantry.

Classic Pantry Oatmeal

Ingredients

- ½ cup rolled oats.
- 1 cup water or shelf-stable or powdered milk.
- 1 tbsp honey or sugar.
- 1 tbsp peanut butter.
- 2 tbsp raisins or dried fruit.
- Pinch of cinnamon.

Instructions

1. Bring the water or milk to a simmer.
2. Add oats and cook for 3–5 minutes.
3. Stir in peanut butter and honey.
4. Sprinkle raisins and cinnamon on top.

Optional Add-ins

- Canned peaches or apples.
- Chopped nuts.
- Coconut flakes.

My Notes...

Peanut Butter Honey Oatmeal

Serves: 1

Ingredients

- ½ cup oats
- 1 cup water or shelf-stable or powdered milk
- 2 tbsp peanut butter
- 1 tbsp honey
- Pinch salt

Instructions

1. Cook oats in water or milk until soft.
2. Stir in peanut butter and honey.
3. Mix until creamy and serve warm.

My Notes...

Apple Cinnamon Oatmeal

Serves: 1

Ingredients

- ½ cup rolled oats
- 1 cup water or shelf-stable or powdered milk
- ½ cup canned apples (or applesauce)
- 1 tbsp brown sugar or honey
- ¼ tsp cinnamon
- Pinch salt

Instructions

1. Bring water or milk to a simmer in a small saucepan.
2. Add oats and salt. Cook for about 3–5 minutes.
3. Stir in canned apples and cinnamon.
4. Sweeten with brown sugar or honey before serving.

My Notes...

Maple Raisin Oatmeal

Serves: 1

Ingredients

- ½ cup rolled oats
- 1 cup water or shelf-stable or powdered milk
- 2 tbsp raisins
- 1 tbsp maple syrup or honey
- Pinch cinnamon

Instructions

1. Bring water or milk to a simmer.
2. Add oats and cook for 3–5 minutes.
3. Stir in raisins and maple syrup.
4. Sprinkle with cinnamon before serving.

My Notes...

Peanut Butter Breakfast Toast Substitute

Serves: 1

Ingredients

- Crackers or crispbread
- 2 tbsp peanut butter
- 1 tbsp honey
- Sprinkle cinnamon

Instructions

1. Spread peanut butter on crackers.
2. Drizzle honey on top.
3. Sprinkle with cinnamon.

Variation: Add sliced canned bananas or dried fruit.

My Notes...

Peanut Butter Banana Breakfast Bowl

Ingredients

- ½ cup oats or granola
- ¾ cup shelf-stable or powdered milk
- 2 tbsp peanut butter
- ½ cup canned bananas or dried banana chips
- 1 tsp honey

Instructions

1. Place oats or granola in a bowl.
2. Pour milk over the oats.
3. Add peanut butter and banana.
4. Drizzle honey on top and mix gently.

My Notes...

Peanut Butter Energy Bowl

Serves: 1

Ingredients

- ½ cup granola or oats
- 2 tbsp peanut butter
- 2 tbsp raisins or dried fruit
- 1 tbsp honey
- ½ cup shelf-stable or powdered milk (optional)

Instructions

1. Place granola or oats in a bowl.
2. Add peanut butter and dried fruit.
3. Drizzle honey on top.
4. Add milk if desired and mix together.

Tip: This meal provides **quick energy and protein**.

My Notes

Creamy Rice Breakfast Bowl

Serves: 2

Ingredients

- 1 cup cooked rice
- 1 cup shelf-stable milk or evaporated milk diluted with water
- 2 tbsp sugar or honey
- ¼ tsp cinnamon
- ¼ cup raisins or dried cranberries

Instructions

1. Combine rice and milk in a saucepan.
2. Warm over medium heat.
3. Stir in sugar, cinnamon, and dried fruit.
4. Simmer until creamy.

My Notes...

Sweet Couscous Breakfast Bowl

Serves: 2

Ingredients

- 1 cup couscous
- 1 cup boiling water
- 2 tbsp honey
- ¼ cup dried fruit
- 2 tbsp nuts or seeds
- Pinch cinnamon

Instructions

1. Pour boiling water over couscous and cover.
2. Let sit 5 minutes.
3. Fluff with a fork.
4. Stir in honey, fruit, nuts, and cinnamon.

My Notes...

Chocolate Oat Breakfast Bowl

Serves: 1

Ingredients

- ½ cup oats
- 1 cup milk or water
- 1 tbsp cocoa powder
- 1 tbsp sugar or honey
- 1 tbsp peanut butter

Instructions

1. Cook oats in milk or water.
2. Stir in cocoa powder and sugar.
3. Add peanut butter and mix well.

My Notes...

Breakfast Muesli Bowl

Serves: 2

Ingredients

- 1 cup oats
- 2 tbsp honey
- 2 tbsp peanut butter
- ¼ cup dried fruit
- 2 tbsp nuts or seeds (optional)

Instructions

1. Mix oats, honey, and peanut butter.
2. Spread on a baking tray.
3. Bake at 175°C (350°F) for 10–15 minutes until toasted.
4. Stir in dried fruit and nuts.

Serve with **powdered milk or shelf-stable milk**.

My Notes...

Pantry Muesli Bars

Ingredients

- 2 cups oats
- ½ cup peanut butter
- ⅓ cup honey
- ¼ cup dried fruit
- ¼ cup nuts or seeds

Instructions

1. Mix peanut butter and honey until smooth.
2. Stir in oats, fruit, and nuts.
3. Press mixture into a lined pan.
4. Refrigerate for 1 hour and cut into bars.

My Notes...

Pantry Pancakes

Serves: 3–4

Ingredients

- 1 cup flour
- 1 tbsp sugar
- 1 tsp baking powder
- Pinch salt
- 1 cup powdered milk mixed with water
- 1 tbsp oil
- ½ tsp vanilla (optional)

Instructions

1. Mix flour, sugar, baking powder, and salt.
2. Add milk mixture and oil.
3. Stir until smooth.
4. Cook in a lightly oiled pan until bubbles form, then flip.

My Notes...

Honey Almond Breakfast Couscous

Serves: 2

Ingredients

- 1 cup couscous
- 1 cup boiling water
- 2 tbsp honey
- ¼ cup raisins
- 2 tbsp almonds or other nuts
- ¼ tsp cinnamon

Instructions

1. Place couscous in a bowl and pour boiling water over it.
2. Cover and let sit for 5 minutes.
3. Fluff with a fork.
4. Stir in honey, raisins, nuts, and cinnamon.

My Notes...

Cinnamon Breakfast Quinoa

Serves: 2

Ingredients

- 1 cup cooked quinoa
- ¾ cup shelf-stable milk
- 2 tbsp honey or sugar
- ¼ tsp cinnamon
- 2 tbsp dried cranberries or raisins

Instructions

1. Combine quinoa and milk in a saucepan.
2. Heat gently while stirring.
3. Add honey, cinnamon, and dried fruit.
4. Serve warm.

My Notes...

Simple Breakfast Polenta

Ingredients

- ½ cup cornmeal
- 2 cups water
- 2 tbsp honey or maple syrup
- Pinch salt
- 2 tbsp dried fruit

Instructions

1. Bring water and salt to a boil.
2. Slowly whisk in cornmeal.
3. Cook 5–7 minutes until thick.
4. Stir in honey and dried fruit.

My Notes...

Emergency Breakfast Mug Cake

Serves: 1

Ingredients

- 4 tbsp flour
- 1 tbsp sugar
- ¼ tsp baking powder
- 3 tbsp powdered milk mixture
- 1 tbsp oil
- 1 tbsp peanut butter

Instructions

1. Mix all ingredients in a mug.
2. Microwave 60–90 seconds.
3. Let cool slightly before eating.

My Notes...

Pantry Breakfast Smoothie (No Fresh Fruit)

Serves: 1

Ingredients

- 1 cup shelf-stable milk or powdered milk mixture
- 2 tbsp peanut butter
- 2 tbsp oats
- 2 tbsp canned fruit or applesauce
- 1 tsp honey

Instructions

1. Combine all ingredients in a blender.
2. Blend until smooth.
3. Serve immediately.

My Notes...

Simple Pantry Muffins

Makes: 6 muffins

Ingredients

- 1 cup flour
- ⅓ cup sugar
- 1 tsp baking powder
- ½ cup powdered milk mixture
- 2 tbsp oil
- ½ cup raisins or dried fruit

Instructions

1. Preheat oven to **350°F (175°C)**.
2. Mix flour, sugar, and baking powder.
3. Stir in milk mixture and oil.
4. Fold in raisins.
5. Pour into muffin tin and bake **15–18 minutes**.

My Notes...

Honey Peanut Butter Crackers

Serves: 1

Ingredients

- 6–8 whole-grain crackers
- 2 tbsp peanut butter
- 1 tbsp honey
- 2 tbsp dried fruit

Instructions

1. Spread peanut butter on crackers.
2. Drizzle honey over the peanut butter.
3. Sprinkle dried fruit on top.

Tip: This is a quick, filling breakfast with protein and healthy fats.

My Notes...

Breakfast Rice with Coconut Milk

Serves: 2

Ingredients

- 1 cup cooked rice
- ¾ cup canned coconut milk
- 2 tbsp sugar or honey
- ¼ cup raisins
- Pinch cinnamon

Instructions

1. Heat rice and coconut milk in a saucepan.
2. Stir in sugar and raisins.
3. Cook until warm and creamy.
4. Sprinkle cinnamon on top.

My Notes...

No-Cook Breakfast Trail Mix

Serves: 1–2

Ingredients

- ½ cup nuts (almonds, peanuts, or mixed nuts)
- ¼ cup dried fruit
- ¼ cup granola or cereal
- 2 tbsp chocolate chips (optional)

Instructions

1. Combine all ingredients in a bowl or container.
2. Mix well.
3. Eat as is or serve with shelf-stable milk.

Optional: Add coconut flakes or sunflower seeds.

My Notes...

Savoury Oatmeal with Beans

Serves: 2

Ingredients

- 1 cup cooked oats
- ½ cup canned black beans
- 1 tbsp olive oil
- ½ tsp garlic powder
- Salt and pepper

Instructions

1. Heat olive oil in a pan.
2. Add beans and garlic powder.
3. Stir in cooked oats.
4. Season with salt and pepper.

My Notes...

Savoury Breakfast Rice

Serves: 2

Ingredients

- 1 cup cooked rice
- 1 small can mushrooms, drained
- 1 tbsp olive oil
- ½ tsp garlic powder
- ½ tsp onion powder
- Salt and pepper to taste

Instructions

1. Heat olive oil in a pan.
2. Add mushrooms and cook for 2–3 minutes.
3. Stir in rice and seasonings.
4. Cook until heated through.

Optional: Add canned chicken or tuna for extra protein.

My Notes...

Lunch

Lunch is often a meal that needs to be quick, satisfying, and easy to prepare. When your pantry is stocked with a few reliable staples, it becomes surprisingly simple to create nourishing midday meals without relying on fresh ingredients.

Pantry lunches can be made from foods that store well and are always ready when you need them—beans, rice, pasta, lentils, canned fish, grains, and preserved vegetables. These ingredients are versatile, affordable, and can be combined in countless ways to create filling meals.

The recipes in this section focus on simplicity and convenience. Many require minimal preparation and only basic kitchen equipment, making them ideal for busy days, working from home, camping trips, or times when fresh groceries are not available.

From warm soups and hearty grain bowls to simple pasta dishes and protein-rich bean meals, these recipes are designed to keep you energized through the day while making the most of the foods already in your pantry.

With a little creativity and a few dependable staples, lunchtime can always be both easy and satisfying.

Pantry Tomato Soup

Serves: 2

Ingredients

- 1 can diced tomatoes
- 1 cup water or broth powder mixed with water
- ½ tsp garlic powder
- ½ tsp onion powder
- Salt and pepper

Instructions

1. Combine ingredients in a pot.
2. Simmer for 10 minutes.
3. Blend if a smooth soup is desired.

Your Notes...

Simple Lentil Soup

Serves: 3

Ingredients

- 1 cup dried lentils
- 4 cups water or broth
- 1 tsp garlic powder
- ½ tsp cumin
- Salt and pepper

Instructions

1. Combine all ingredients in a pot.
2. Simmer 20–25 minutes until lentils are tender.

Your Notes...

Tuna & Bean Salad

Serves: 2

Ingredients

- 1 can tuna
- 1 can white beans, drained
- 1 tbsp olive oil
- 1 tbsp vinegar or lemon juice
- ½ tsp garlic powder
- Salt and pepper

Instructions

1. Combine tuna and beans in a bowl.
2. Add oil, vinegar, garlic powder, salt, and pepper.
3. Toss gently and serve.

Your Notes...

Chickpea Salad Bowl

Serves: 2

Ingredients

- 1 can chickpeas
- 1 tbsp olive oil
- 1 tbsp vinegar
- ½ tsp paprika
- Salt and pepper

Instructions

1. Drain chickpeas.
2. Toss with oil, vinegar, paprika, salt, and pepper.

Your Notes...

Peanut Noodle Bowl

Serves: 2

Ingredients

- 200 g dried noodles
- 2 tbsp peanut butter
- 1 tbsp soy sauce
- 1 tsp honey
- Chili flakes (optional)

Instructions

1. Cook noodles according to package instructions.
2. Mix peanut butter, soy sauce, and honey.
3. Toss noodles with sauce.

Your Notes...

Rice & Beans Lunch Bowl

Serves: 2

Ingredients

- 1 cup cooked rice
- 1 can black beans
- 1 tsp cumin
- 1 tbsp olive oil
- Salt and pepper

Instructions

1. Heat beans with cumin.
2. Serve over rice with olive oil.

Your Notes...

Canned Chicken Rice Bowl

Serves: 2

Ingredients

- 1 cup rice
- 1 can of chicken
- 1 tsp garlic powder
- 1 tbsp olive oil
- Salt and pepper

Instructions

1. Heat rice and chicken together.
2. Season with garlic powder, oil, salt, and pepper.

Your Notes...

Couscous Vegetable Bowl

Serves: 2

Ingredients

- 1 cup couscous
- 1 cup boiling water
- ½ cup canned corn
- 1 tbsp olive oil
- Salt and pepper

Instructions

1. Pour boiling water over couscous.
2. Let sit 5 minutes.
3. Stir in corn and olive oil.

Your Notes...

Bean & Rice Burrito Bowl

Serves: 2

Preparation Time: About 10 minutes

Ingredients

- 1 cup cooked rice (white or brown)
- 1 can beans, drained and rinsed (black beans, kidney beans, or pinto beans work well)
- ½ cup canned corn, drained
- 1 teaspoon chilli powder
- ½ teaspoon ground cumin (optional)
- Salt and pepper to taste

Instructions

1. Cook the rice according to package instructions if it is not already prepared.
2. In a small saucepan, combine the beans and corn. Heat gently over medium heat for 3–5 minutes until warmed through.
3. Stir in the chili powder, cumin (if using), and a pinch of salt and pepper.
4. Divide the cooked rice between two bowls.
5. Spoon the seasoned bean and corn mixture over the rice.
6. Add any optional toppings you have available.

Savoury Oatmeal Bowl

Serves: 1–2

Preparation Time: About 10 minutes

Ingredients

- 1 cup rolled oats or quick oats
- 2 cups water or broth
- ½ cup canned beans, drained and rinsed (black beans, kidney beans, or chickpeas)
- 1 tablespoon olive oil
- Salt and black pepper to taste

Instructions

1. In a small saucepan, bring the water or broth to a gentle boil.
2. Add the oats and reduce the heat to medium-low.
3. Cook for about 5 minutes, stirring occasionally, until the oats are soft and creamy.
4. Stir in the beans and cook for another minute until warmed through.
5. Spoon the oatmeal into bowls and drizzle with olive oil.
6. Season with salt and black pepper to taste.
7. Add any optional toppings you have available.

Chickpea Curry Bowl

Serves: 2

Preparation Time: About 15 minutes

Ingredients

- 1 cup cooked rice (white or brown)
- 1 can chickpeas, drained and rinsed
- ½ cup coconut milk (or about half a can)
- 1 teaspoon curry powder
- ½ teaspoon garlic powder or minced garlic (optional)
- Salt and black pepper to taste

Instructions

1. Cook the rice according to package instructions if it is not already prepared.
2. In a small saucepan or skillet, add the chickpeas and coconut milk.
3. Stir in the curry powder and garlic powder if using.
4. Bring the mixture to a gentle simmer over medium heat.
5. Let it cook for about 5–8 minutes, stirring occasionally, until the sauce thickens slightly and the chickpeas are heated through.
6. Season with salt and pepper to taste.

Tomato Couscous Soup

Serves: 2

Ingredients

- 1 can diced tomatoes (about 400 g / 14 oz)
- 2 cups vegetable or chicken broth
- ½ cup couscous
- ½ teaspoon garlic powder or minced garlic (optional)
- ½ teaspoon dried oregano or basil
- Salt and black pepper to taste
- 1 tablespoon olive oil (optional)

Instructions

1. In a medium saucepan, combine the canned tomatoes and broth.
2. Add the garlic powder, oregano or basil, and a pinch of salt and pepper.
3. Bring the mixture to a gentle boil over medium heat.
4. Stir in the couscous and reduce the heat slightly.
5. Let the soup simmer for about 8–10 minutes until the couscous is tender.
6. Stir in olive oil if using, and adjust seasoning to taste.
7. Ladle the soup into bowls and add any optional toppings.

Creamy Pantry Pasta

Serves: 3

Ingredients

- 250 g pasta
- 1 can evaporated milk
- ½ tsp garlic powder
- ½ tsp onion powder
- Your Favourite Spices and Herbs
- Salt and pepper

Instructions

1. Cook pasta.
2. Heat milk with seasonings.
3. Stir pasta into the sauce.

Your Notes...

Tomato & Bean Stew

Serves: 3

Ingredients

- 1 can of kidney beans
- 1 can of tomatoes
- 1 tsp paprika
- ½ tsp garlic powder
- Salt and pepper

Instructions

1. Combine all ingredients in a pot.
2. Simmer 15 minutes.

Your Notes...

Lentil Tomato Stew

Serves: 2–3

Ingredients

- 1 cup dried lentils (red, brown, or green), rinsed
- 1 can diced tomatoes (about 400 g / 14 oz)
- 2 cups water or vegetable broth
- 1 teaspoon garlic powder
- 1 teaspoon ground cumin
- ½ teaspoon paprika (optional)
- Salt and black pepper to taste
- 1 tablespoon olive oil (optional)

Instructions

1. Rinse the lentils under cold water and remove any debris.
2. In a pot, combine lentils, tomatoes, and water or broth.
3. Add the garlic powder, cumin, paprika (if using), and a pinch of salt and pepper.
4. Bring the mixture to a gentle boil over medium heat.
5. Reduce the heat to low and let the stew simmer until the lentils are tender.
6. If the stew becomes too thick, add a little extra water or broth.
7. Stir in olive oil if using, adjust seasoning to taste, and add any optional ingredients before serving.

Tuna Pasta Salad

Serves: 3

Preparation Time: About 15 minutes

Ingredients

- 2 cups cooked pasta (any small pasta such as macaroni, penne, or shells)
- 1 can tuna, drained
- ½ cup canned corn, drained
- 1–2 tablespoons olive oil
- ½ teaspoon garlic powder
- Salt and black pepper to taste

Instructions

1. Cook the pasta according to package instructions. Drain and allow it to cool slightly.
2. Place the cooked pasta in a large bowl.
3. Add the drained tuna and canned corn.
4. Drizzle with olive oil and sprinkle with garlic powder, salt, and pepper.
5. Gently mix everything together until well combined.
6. Taste and adjust seasoning as needed.
7. Add any optional ingredients you have available and mix again before serving.

Peanut Butter Ramen

Serves: 1–2

Preparation Time: About 10 minutes

Ingredients

- 1 packet instant ramen noodles (discard or reduce the seasoning packet if desired)
- 1½ cups water
- 1–2 tablespoons peanut butter
- 1–2 teaspoons soy sauce
- ½ teaspoon garlic powder (optional)
- A pinch of chilli flakes or hot sauce (optional)

Instructions

1. Bring the water to a boil in a small saucepan.
2. Add the ramen noodles and cook according to the package instructions, usually about 3–4 minutes.
3. Stir in the peanut butter and soy sauce until the peanut butter melts and creates a creamy sauce.
4. Add garlic powder and chilli flakes if using.
5. Add any optional vegetables or protein and cook briefly until heated through.
6. Serve warm and garnish with any optional toppings.

Bread and Damper Recipes

Bread has been a staple food for thousands of years, made from some of the simplest ingredients found in almost every kitchen. Flour, water, salt, and a little fat or leavening can be transformed into warm, comforting bread that pairs perfectly with soups, stews, and spreads.

In times when fresh groceries are limited, knowing how to make bread from pantry staples can be especially valuable. With ingredients that store well—such as flour, baking powder, yeast, oil, powdered milk, and dried herbs—you can create a variety of satisfying breads without needing fresh items.

One of the most well-known pantry breads is **damper**, a traditional Australian bread once cooked by stockmen and travellers over campfires. Made from only a few basic ingredients, damper is a wonderful example of how simple foods can still be hearty and delicious. Today it can be baked in an oven, cooked in a skillet, or even prepared over an open fire.

The recipes in this section are designed to be practical and approachable. From quick flatbreads and soda breads to classic damper and simple yeast loaves, each recipe uses ingredients that are easy to store and keep on hand. Many require minimal preparation and only basic kitchen equipment.

Freshly baked bread has a way of bringing comfort and warmth to the table. Even the simplest meal can feel more complete when served with a piece of homemade bread. With these easy pantry recipes, you'll always be able to create something wholesome and satisfying from the ingredients already in your cupboard.

Your Notes....

Traditional Campfire Damper

Serves: 4

Ingredients

- 3 cups self-raising flour
- 1 tsp salt
- 1 tbsp of oil
- 1 cup water or powdered milk mixture

Instructions

1. Mix flour and salt.
2. Add oil and water, knead to form dough.
3. Shape into a round loaf.
4. Bake **30 minutes at 180°C / 350°F**.

Your Notes...

Simple Oven Damper

Serves: 4

Ingredients

- 3 cups self-raising flour
- 1 tsp sugar
- 1 cup shelf-stable milk (powdered milk mix)
- 1 tbsp of oil

Instructions

1. Mix flour and sugar.
2. Add milk and oil.
3. Shape into dough and bake **30 minutes at 180°C / 350°F**.

Your Notes...

Quick Flatbread

Serves: 4

Ingredients

- 2 cups flour
- 1 tsp salt
- 1 tbsp oil
- ¾ cup water

Instructions

1. Mix ingredients to form dough.
2. Divide into balls.
3. Roll flat and cook in a hot pan 2–3 minutes per side.

Your Notes...

Pantry Soda Bread

Serves: 6

Ingredients

- 3 cups flour
- 1 tsp baking soda
- 1 tsp salt
- 1½ cups powdered milk mixture

Instructions

1. Mix dry ingredients.
2. Add milk and form dough.
3. Bake **35 minutes at 180°C / 350°F**.

Your Notes...

Basic Pantry Yeast Bread

Makes: 1 loaf

Ingredients

- 3 cups flour
- 1 tsp salt
- 1 tbsp sugar
- 2 tsp dry yeast
- 1 tbsp oil
- 1 cup warm water

Instructions

1. Mix warm water, sugar, and yeast. Let it sit for 5 minutes.
2. Add flour, salt, and oil.
3. Knead for about 8 minutes.
4. Let rise for 1 hour.
5. Shape into a loaf and bake **30 minutes at 180°C / 350°F**.

Your Notes...

Quick Skillet Bread

Ingredients

- 2 cups flour
- 1 tsp baking powder
- 1 tsp salt
- 1 tbsp oil
- ¾ cup water

Instructions

1. Mix all ingredients into a dough.
2. Divide into 6 balls.
3. Flatten into circles.
4. Your NoCook in a hot skillet for 3–4 minutes per side.

Your Notes...

Savoury Herb Soda Bread

Serves: 6

Ingredients

- 3 cups flour
- 1 tsp baking soda
- 1 tsp salt
- 1 tbsp dried herbs
- 1½ cups powdered milk mixture

Instructions

1. Mix dry ingredients.
2. Add milk mixture to form dough.
3. Shape into a round loaf.
4. Bake **35 minutes at 180°C / 350°F**.

Your Notes...

Honey Oat Bread

Makes: 1 loaf

Ingredients

- 2 cups flour
- 1 cup oats
- 1 tbsp honey
- 1 tsp salt
- 2 tsp yeast
- 1¼ cups warm water

Instructions

1. Combine yeast and warm water.
2. Add remaining ingredients and mix into a dough.
3. Knead until smooth.
4. Let rise 1 hour.
5. Bake **30–35 minutes at 180°C / 350°F**.

Your Notes...

Sweet Raisin Bread

Makes: 1 loaf

Ingredients

- 3 cups flour
- 2 tbsp sugar
- 1 tsp salt
- 2 tsp yeast
- 1 cup warm water
- ½ cup raisins
- 1 tsp cinnamon

Instructions

1. Mix yeast with warm water.
2. Add flour, sugar, salt, and cinnamon.
3. Stir in raisins.
4. Let rise 1 hour.
5. Bake **30 minutes at 180°C / 350°F**.

Raisins can be substituted with other dried fruits.

Your Notes...

Simple Fry Bread

Makes: 6 pieces

Ingredients

- 2 cups flour
- 1 tsp baking powder
- 1 tsp salt
- ¾ cup water
- Oil for frying

Instructions

1. Mix flour, baking powder, salt, and water.
2. Divide the dough into balls and flatten.
3. Fry in hot oil until golden.

Your Notes...

Simple Cornbread

Serves: 6

Ingredients

- 1 cup cornmeal
- 1 cup flour
- 2 tsp baking powder
- ¼ cup sugar
- 1 cup powdered milk mixture
- 2 tbsp oil

Instructions

1. Mix all ingredients together.
2. Pour into a greased pan.
3. Bake **20–25 minutes at 180°C / 350°F**.

Your Notes...

Soft Dinner Rolls

Makes: 8 rolls

Ingredients

- 3 cups flour
- 1 tbsp sugar
- 1 tsp salt
- 2 tsp yeast
- 1 cup warm water
- 2 tbsp oil

Instructions

1. Mix yeast with warm water and sugar.
2. Add flour, salt, and oil.
3. Knead and let rise 1 hour.
4. Shape into rolls.
5. Bake **18–20 minutes at 180°C / 350°F**.

Your Notes...

Simple Crackers

Ingredients

- 1 cup flour
- ½ tsp salt
- 2 tbsp oil
- ¼ cup water

Instructions

1. Mix the dough and roll it thin.
2. Cut into squares.
3. Bake **12–15 minutes at 180°C / 350°F**.

Your Notes...

Pantry Flour Tortillas

Ingredients

- 2 cups plain flour
- ½ tsp salt
- 1 tsp baking powder *(optional, but makes them softer)*
- 2 tbsp oil *(olive oil, vegetable oil, or melted shortening)*
- ¾ cup warm water

Instructions

1. Mix dry ingredients

   In a bowl, combine flour, salt, and baking powder.
2. Add oil.
3. Add water
4. Knead.
5. Rest the dough

   Cover and let rest 10–15 minutes (this makes rolling easier).
6. Divide

   Cut the dough into 8 small balls.
7. Roll each ball into a thin circle
8. Cook in a frying pan over **medium-high heat**.

   Cook each tortilla for **30–45 seconds**

Garlic Herb Flatbread

Makes: 6 pieces

Ingredients

- 2 cups flour
- 1 tsp salt
- 1 tsp garlic powder
- 1 tsp dried herbs
- 1 tbsp olive oil
- ¾ cup water

Instructions

1. Mix ingredients into the dough.
2. Divide and roll flat.
3. Cook in a skillet until golden.

Your Notes...

Hardtack (Long-Lasting Survival Bread)

Makes: about 12 crackers

Ingredients

- 2 cups flour
- 1 tsp salt
- ¾ cup water

Instructions

1. Mix ingredients into stiff dough.
2. Roll thin and cut into squares.
3. Poke holes with a fork.
4. Bake **30 minutes at 180°C / 350°F**, turning halfway.

Tip: Hardtack stores for **months when kept dry**.

Bean Bread Recipes

For generations, women have turned simple pantry staples into sustaining meals. Long before modern grocery stores and food delivery, families relied on dried beans, stored grains, and preserved ingredients. Bean breads emerged from that necessity—hearty, protein-rich loaves that could stretch limited supplies and keep a household fed.

Beans transform humble bread into something far more nourishing. They add protein, fibre, and a satisfying density that keeps hunger away longer than simple flour breads. In times when fresh ingredients are scarce—during winter, economic hardship, or emergencies—bean breads become a quiet form of resilience.

What makes them especially valuable is that most recipes rely on foods that store well for months or even years: dried or canned beans, baking powder, salt, oil, and shelf-stable grains. With little more than a bowl and a baking pan, a nourishing loaf can emerge from the pantry.

Bean breads are also endlessly adaptable. Different cultures have created their own versions—from savoury loaves made with white beans and herbs to sweet breads using black beans and cocoa. Each variation reflects creativity born from necessity.

Rustic White Bean Skillet Bread

A dense, savoury bread that pairs well with soup.

Ingredients

- 1 cup mashed canned white beans (drained)
- 1 cup flour (or oat flour)
- 1 tsp baking powder
- ½ tsp salt
- 1 tbsp olive oil
- ½ cup water or milk powder reconstituted
- Optional: dried rosemary or garlic powder

Instructions

1. Preheat oven to **190°C (375°F)**.
2. Mash beans until mostly smooth.
3. Mix flour, baking powder, salt, and herbs.
4. Stir in beans, oil, and liquid to form a thick batter.
5. Spread into a greased skillet or small pan.
6. Bake **25–30 minutes** until firm and lightly browned.

Your Notes...

Black Bean Pantry Bread (High Protein)

A surprisingly rich bread made almost entirely from beans.

Ingredients

- 1 can black beans, drained
- 2 eggs (or powdered eggs)
- 2 tbsp oil
- ¼ cup cocoa powder
- ¼ cup sugar or honey
- 1 tsp baking powder
- pinch of salt

Instructions

1. Blend all ingredients until smooth.
2. Pour into a greased loaf pan.
3. Bake **30 minutes at 175°C (350°F)**.

Result: a soft, brownie-like bread high in protein.

Your Notes...

Chickpea Flatbread

Inspired by traditional Mediterranean and Indian pantry cooking.

Ingredients

- 1 cup chickpea flour (or ground dried chickpeas)
- 1 cup water
- ½ tsp salt
- 1 tbsp oil

Instructions

1. Mix ingredients into a thin batter.
2. Heat a lightly oiled skillet.
3. Pour batter and cook like a pancake.
4. Flip when edges crisp.

This bread requires **no yeast and no fresh ingredients**, making it perfect for pantry cooking.

Your Notes...

Sweet Bean Bread

A comforting loaf when fresh ingredients are limited.

Ingredients

- 1 cup mashed navy beans
- ¾ cup flour
- ½ cup sugar or maple syrup
- 1 tsp cinnamon
- 1 tsp baking powder
- ¼ cup oil
- ½ cup water

Instructions

1. Mix wet ingredients with mashed beans.
2. Add dry ingredients.
3. Bake 40 minutes at 350°F.

This bread resembles a soft spice loaf.

Making Pasta from Pantry Ingredients

Pasta is one of the most useful and versatile foods in the pantry. It stores well for long periods and can be used in a wide variety of meals. However, if dried pasta is unavailable, it is still possible to make simple pasta using basic ingredients that are commonly found in many kitchens.

Traditional pasta requires only a few ingredients—typically flour, eggs, and water. In situations where fresh eggs are not available, pasta can also be made using just flour and water, or by using shelf-stable alternatives such as powdered eggs.

Homemade pasta does not require special equipment. The dough can be mixed by hand, rolled out with a rolling pin, and cut into simple shapes using a knife. Once prepared, fresh pasta cooks quickly in boiling water and can be used in soups, sauces, or simple pantry meals.

The following recipes show a few easy ways to prepare pasta using ingredients that store well in the pantry.

Tips for Homemade Pantry Pasta

- If the dough feels sticky, add a little more flour.
- If the dough is too dry, add a small amount of water.
- Fresh pasta cooks much faster than dried pasta.
- Pasta can be added directly to soups, stews, or sauces.

Basic Flour and Water Pasta

This is one of the simplest forms of pasta and requires only two ingredients.

Ingredients

2 cups plain flour

¾ cup water

½ tsp salt (optional)

Instructions

1. Place flour and salt in a bowl.
2. Gradually add water while mixing until a dough forms.
3. Knead the dough on a floured surface for about 5–10 minutes until smooth.
4. Cover and let the dough rest for 15 minutes.
5. Roll the dough thin with a rolling pin.
6. Cut into strips or small squares using a knife.
7. Cook in boiling water for 3–5 minutes.

Your Notes...

Pantry Egg Pasta (Using Powdered Eggs)

Ingredients

2 cups flour

2 tbsp powdered egg

½ cup water

½ tsp salt

Instructions

1. Mix flour, powdered egg, and salt in a bowl.
2. Add water gradually while mixing.
3. Knead dough for 5–10 minutes until smooth.
4. Let the dough rest for 15 minutes.
5. Roll thin and cut into noodles.
6. Cook in boiling water for 3–4 minutes.

Your Notes...

Simple Dumpling-Style Pasta

This method is quick and requires no rolling.

Ingredients

1 cup flour

½ cup water

½ tsp salt

Instructions

1. Mix flour, salt, and water to form a thick dough.
2. Bring a pot of water or soup to a gentle boil.
3. Drop small spoonfuls of dough into the boiling liquid.
4. Cook for 3–5 minutes until firm.

This style works well in soups and stews.

Your Notes...

Flat Survival Noodles

These noodles are easy to make and require very little equipment.

Ingredients

2 cups flour

¾ cup water

½ tsp salt

Instructions

1. Mix ingredients into a dough.
2. Knead until smooth.
3. Roll the dough thin.
4. Cut into wide strips using a knife.
5. Cook in boiling water for about 4 minutes.

Your Notes...

Pantry Dinner Recipes

Dinner is often the meal we look forward to most at the end of a long day. It brings comfort, warmth, and the chance to gather around the table. Even when fresh ingredients are limited, a well-stocked pantry can provide everything needed to create satisfying evening meals.

Pantry cooking is about creativity and practicality. Canned beans, lentils, rice, pasta, grains, and preserved vegetables can be transformed into nourishing dishes with just a few herbs and spices. These recipes are designed to make the most of foods that store well and are easy to keep on hand.

Whether you are preparing meals during a busy week, stretching your grocery budget, cooking while camping, or managing during a power outage or emergency situation, pantry meals can still be hearty, flavourful, and comforting.

The recipes in this section focus on simple ingredients and straightforward cooking methods. Many can be prepared in a single pot and require only basic kitchen equipment. They are filling, affordable, and designed to help you turn everyday pantry staples into delicious dinners for yourself, your family, or anyone gathered around your table.

Tomato Bean Soup

Serves: 3

Preparation Time: About 20 minutes

Ingredients

- 1 can diced tomatoes (about 400 g / 14 oz)
- 1 can white beans (such as cannellini, navy beans, or great northern beans), drained and rinsed
- 2 cups vegetable or chicken broth
- ½–1 teaspoon garlic powder
- ½ teaspoon dried oregano or basil (optional)
- Salt and black pepper to taste
- 1 tablespoon olive oil (optional)

Instructions

1. In a medium saucepan, combine the canned tomatoes, white beans, and broth.
2. Add the garlic, your favourite herbs and spices, oregano or basil if using, and a pinch of salt and pepper.
3. Bring the mixture to a gentle boil over medium heat.
4. Simmer for about 15 minutes, stirring occasionally.
5. Stir in olive oil if using and adjust the seasoning to taste.
6. Add any optional ingredients during the last few minutes of cooking.

Pantry Vegetable Soup

Serves: 4

Preparation Time: About 25 minutes

Ingredients

- 1 can diced tomatoes
- 1 can mixed vegetables
- 1 can of beans drained and rinsed
- 3 cups vegetable or chicken broth
- 2 teaspoons dried herbs
- 1 teaspoon garlic powder
- Salt and black pepper to taste
- 1 tablespoon olive oil (optional)

Instructions

1. In a large saucepan or pot, combine the canned tomatoes, canned vegetables, beans, and broth.
2. Add the dried herbs, garlic powder, salt, and pepper.
3. Bring the soup to a gentle boil over medium heat.
4. Simmer for about 15–20 minutes
5. If using pasta, rice, or barley, stir it in during the simmering stage and cook until tender.
6. Stir in olive oil if desired and adjust seasoning to taste.
7. Serve warm and add any optional toppings if available.

Simple Curry Chickpea Soup

Serves: 3–4

Ingredients

- 1 can chickpeas
- 1 can of tomatoes
- 2 cups broth or water
- 2 tbsp curry powder
- 1 tsp garlic powder

Instructions

1. Combine all ingredients in a pot.
2. Simmer **15 minutes** for a light curry soup.

Your Notes...

Hearty Pantry Chilli

Serves: 4

Ingredients

- 1 can of kidney beans
- 1 can black beans
- 1 can diced tomatoes
- 1 small can of corn
- 1 tsp chilli powder
- ½ tsp cumin
- Salt and pepper

Instructions

1. Combine all ingredients in a pot.
2. Simmer for 20 minutes.
3. Serve with bread or rice.

Your Notes....

Simple Lentil Stew

Serves: 3

Ingredients

- 1 cup dried lentils
- 4 cups water or broth
- 1 can of tomatoes
- 1 tsp garlic powder
- ½ tsp cumin

Instructions

1. Combine all ingredients in a pot.
2. Simmer 25–30 minutes until lentils soften.

Your Notes...

Chickpea Tomato Stew

Serves: 3

Ingredients

- 1 can chickpeas, drained and rinsed
- 1 can diced tomatoes
- 1½ cups vegetable or chicken broth
- 1 teaspoon garlic powder
- 1 teaspoon paprika
- ½ teaspoon ground cumin (optional)
- Salt and black pepper to taste
- 1 tablespoon olive oil (optional)

Instructions

1. In a medium saucepan or pot, combine the chickpeas, canned tomatoes, and broth.
2. Add the garlic powder, paprika, cumin (if using), and a pinch of salt and black pepper.
3. Bring the mixture to a gentle boil over medium heat.
4. Simmer for about 15 minutes, stirring occasionally.
5. If using additional vegetables, add them during the simmering stage and cook until tender.
6. Stir in olive oil if desired and adjust the seasoning to taste.

Creamy Corn Chowder

Serves: 3

Preparation Time: About 15 minutes

Ingredients

- 1 can corn (about 400 g / 14 oz), drained
- 1 cup evaporated milk
- 1½ cups vegetable or chicken broth
- ½ teaspoon garlic powder
- ½ teaspoon onion powder (optional)
- Salt and black pepper to taste
- 1 tablespoon butter or olive oil (optional)

Instructions

1. In a medium saucepan, combine the canned corn and broth.
2. Add the garlic powder, onion powder if using, and a pinch of salt and pepper.
3. Bring the mixture to a gentle simmer over medium heat.
4. Stir in the evaporated milk and continue to cook for about 8–10 minutes, stirring occasionally.
5. If using potatoes or other vegetables, add them during the simmering stage and cook until heated through.
6. Stir in butter or olive oil if desired for extra richness.

Tomato Lentil Pasta

Serves: 3

Ingredients

- 2 cups cooked pasta (such as penne, macaroni, or shells)
- 1 cup cooked lentils or 1 can lentils, drained and rinsed
- 1 can diced tomatoes
- 1 teaspoon garlic powder
- ½ teaspoon dried oregano or basil (optional)
- Salt and black pepper to taste
- 1 tablespoon olive oil (optional)

Instructions

1. Cook the pasta according to the package instructions.
2. In a saucepan, combine the lentils and canned tomatoes.
3. Add the garlic powder, oregano or basil if using, and a pinch of salt and pepper.
4. Heat the mixture over medium heat and allow it to simmer for about 5–7 minutes so the flavours combine.
5. Stir in olive oil if using and add any optional vegetables during the simmering stage.
6. Add the cooked pasta to the saucepan and gently mix until everything is well combined and heated through.

Tuna Tomato Pasta

Serves: 3

Ingredients

- 250 g pasta
- 1 can of tuna
- 1 can diced tomatoes
- 1 tsp garlic powder
- Salt and pepper

Instructions

1. Cook pasta.
2. Heat tomatoes with garlic powder.
3. Stir in tuna and cooked pasta.

Your Notes...

Creamy Mushroom Pasta

Serves: 3

Ingredients

- 250 g pasta
- 1 can evaporated milk
- 1 can mushrooms
- ½ tsp garlic powder

Instructions

1. Cook pasta.
2. Heat milk and mushrooms.
3. Mix pasta into the sauce.

Your Notes...

Rice and Beans Skillet

Serves: 3

Ingredients

- 1 cup cooked rice
- 1 can black beans
- 1 tbsp olive oil
- 1 tsp cumin and/ or your favourite herbs and spices
- Salt and pepper

Instructions

1. Heat oil in a skillet.
2. Add beans and seasonings.
3. Stir in rice and cook until heated.

Your Notes...

Lentil & Rice Dinner Bowl

Serves: 3

Ingredients

- 1 cup cooked lentils
- 1 cup cooked rice
- 1 tbsp olive oil
- ½ tsp cumin
- 1 tsp garlic powder
- Salt and pepper

Instructions

1. Combine lentils and rice.
2. Add oil and cumin.
3. Heat and serve.

Your Notes...

Pantry Tomato Rice

Serves: 2

Ingredients

- 1 cup rice
- 1 can diced tomatoes
- ½ tsp garlic powder
- 1 tbsp olive oil
- Salt and your favourite herbs and spices

Instructions

1. Cook rice.
2. Heat tomatoes and garlic powder, salt and herbs
3. Stir into the rice with olive oil.

Your Notes...

Quick Chickpea Curry Bowl

Serves: 2

Ingredients

- 1 can chickpeas
- 1 tbsp curry powder
- 1 tbsp olive oil
- ½ cup canned vegetables (optional)
- Salt and pepper

Instructions

1. Heat chickpeas, vegetables, oil, and spices in a pan.
2. Cook for **8–10 minutes**.
3. Serve over rice or couscous.

Your Notes…

Ramen Pantry Bowl

Serves: 2

Ingredients

- 2 packets instant ramen noodles
- 3 cups water or broth
- 1 can chicken, drained
- 1–2 teaspoons soy sauce
- A pinch of chilli flakes
- ½ teaspoon garlic powder (optional)

Instructions

1. In a medium saucepan, bring the water or broth to a boil.
2. Add the ramen noodles and cook according to the package instructions, usually about 3–4 minutes.
3. Stir in the canned chicken, soy sauce, chilli flakes, and garlic powder if using.
4. If adding vegetables, stir them in during the last few minutes of cooking so they heat through.
5. Continue simmering for another 1–2 minutes until the chicken and vegetables are warmed.
6. Taste the broth and adjust seasoning if needed.
7. Divide the noodles and broth between bowls and add any optional toppings before serving.

Couscous Vegetable Dinner

Serves: 2

Preparation Time: About 10 minutes

Ingredients

- 1 cup couscous
- 1 cup boiling water or broth
- 1 cup canned vegetables (such as mixed vegetables, peas, corn, or carrots), drained
- 1 tablespoon olive oil
- Salt and black pepper to taste

Instructions

1. Place the couscous in a heatproof bowl.
2. Pour the boiling water or broth over the couscous.
3. Cover the bowl with a lid or plate and let it sit for about 5 minutes until the liquid is absorbed.
4. Fluff the couscous with a fork to separate the grains.
5. Stir in the canned vegetables and olive oil.
6. Season with salt and black pepper, and add any optional spices or herbs if using.
7. Mix well and serve warm.

Pantry Shepherd's Pie

Serves: 4

Preparation Time: About 30 minutes

Ingredients

- 1 can lentils, drained and rinsed
- 1 can mixed vegetables
- 1 cup instant mashed potatoes
- 1 teaspoon garlic powder
- 1 teaspoon onion powder (or your favourites)
- Salt and black pepper to taste
- 1 tablespoon olive oil or butter (optional)
- 1 cup vegetable or beef broth (optional, for extra flavour)

Instructions

1. Preheat the oven to **180°C / 350°F**.
2. Combine the lentils and mixed vegetables.
3. Stir in the garlic powder, salt, and black pepper.
4. Add in the broth or tomato paste, mix
5. Spread the mixture evenly in a baking dish.
6. Spread the mashed potatoes evenly over the top
7. Bake in the oven for **about 20 minutes**, or until the top is lightly golden and the filling is heated through.

Peanut Noodle Dinner

Serves: 2

Ingredients

- 200 g noodles
- 2 tbsp peanut butter
- 1 tbsp soy sauce
- 1 tsp honey
- Add your favourite spices

Instructions

1. Cook noodles.
2. Mix peanut butter, soy sauce, and honey.
3. Toss noodles with sauce.

Your Notes....

Pantry Fried Rice

Serves: 3

Ingredients

- 2 cups cooked rice (preferably cooled or leftover rice)
- 1 cup canned mixed vegetables drained
- 1–2 tablespoons soy sauce
- 1 tablespoon cooking oil (vegetable, canola, or sesame oil)
- ½ teaspoon garlic powder
- Salt and black pepper to taste

Instructions

1. Heat the oil in a large skillet or frying pan over medium heat.
2. Add the cooked rice and stir gently to separate the grains.
3. Add the canned vegetables and garlic powder, stirring to combine.
4. Cook for about 3–4 minutes, stirring occasionally, until everything is heated through.
5. Stir in the soy sauce and season
6. If using an egg, push the rice to one side of the pan, pour the beaten egg into the empty space, and scramble it before mixing it into the rice.
7. Add any optional ingredients and cook for another minute or two.

Lentil Curry

Serves: 3

Ingredients

- 1 cup dried lentils (red, brown, or green), rinsed
- 1 cup coconut milk
- 2 cups water or vegetable broth
- 1–2 teaspoons curry powder
- ½ teaspoon garlic powder (optional)
- Salt and black pepper to taste
- 1 tablespoon cooking oil (optional)

Instructions

1. Rinse the lentils under cold water and remove any debris.
2. In a medium saucepan, combine the lentils, water or broth, and coconut milk.
3. Add the curry powder, garlic powder if using, and a pinch of salt and pepper.
4. Bring the mixture to a gentle boil over medium heat.
5. Reduce the heat, simmer for about 20 minutes
6. If using additional vegetables or tomatoes, stir them in during the last few minutes of cooking.
7. Add oil if desired for extra richness and adjust seasoning to taste.

Tuna Rice Skillet

Serves: 2

Ingredients

- 2 cups cooked rice (white or brown)
- 1 can tuna, drained
- 1–2 tablespoons olive oil
- ½ teaspoon garlic powder (optional)
- Salt and black pepper to taste

Instructions

1. Heat the olive oil in a skillet or frying pan over medium heat.
2. Add the cooked rice and stir gently to separate the grains.
3. Cook the rice for about 2–3 minutes, stirring occasionally, until warmed through.
4. Add the drained tuna and garlic powder if using.
5. Stir well to combine and continue cooking for another 2–3 minutes.
6. Add any optional vegetables or seasonings and cook until everything is heated through.
7. Season with salt and black pepper to taste.
8. Serve warm.

Your Notes...

Bean & Tomato Casserole

Serves: 4

Preparation Time: About 30–35 minutes

Ingredients

- 1 can kidney beans, drained and rinsed
- 1 can diced tomatoes
- ½ teaspoon garlic powder
- 1 -2 teaspoon dried herbs
- Salt and black pepper to taste
- 1 tablespoon olive oil (optional)

Instructions

1. Preheat the oven to **180°C / 350°F**.
2. In a mixing bowl, combine the kidney beans and canned tomatoes.
3. Stir in the garlic powder, dried herbs, salt, and black pepper.
4. Add optional ingredients such as tomato paste
5. Transfer to a baking dish and spread it evenly.
6. Drizzle olive oil over the top if using.
7. Bake in the oven for **about 25 minutes**, or until the casserole is heated through and slightly thickened.
8. .

Coconut Rice with Chickpeas

Serves: 3

Ingredients

- 1 cup uncooked rice (white or jasmine works well)
- 1 cup coconut milk
- 1 cup water or vegetable broth
- 1 can chickpeas, drained and rinsed
- ½ teaspoon garlic powder (optional)
- ½ teaspoon ground cumin or curry powder (optional)
- Salt and black pepper to taste
- 1 tablespoon olive oil or coconut oil (optional)

Instructions

1. In a medium saucepan, combine the rice, coconut milk, and water or broth.
2. Add the garlic powder, cumin or curry powder if using, and a pinch of salt and pepper.
3. Bring the mixture to a gentle boil over medium heat.
4. Simmer until the liquid is absorbed and the rice is tender.
5. Add chickpeas and cook for another 2–3 minutes
6. If using additional vegetables, add them during the final few minutes of cooking.
7. Stir in oil if desired and adjust seasoning to taste.

Classic Pantry Chickpea Curry

Serves: 3–4

Ingredients

- 1 can chickpeas, drained
- 1 can diced tomatoes
- 1 can coconut milk
- 1 tbsp curry powder
- 1 tsp garlic powder
- ½ tsp cumin
- Salt and pepper

Instructions

1. Combine all ingredients in a saucepan.
2. Bring to a gentle simmer.
3. Cook for **10–15 minutes**, stirring occasionally.
4. Serve over rice.

Your Notes...

Chickpea Coconut Curry

Serves: 3

Ingredients

- 1 can chickpeas
- 1 can coconut milk
- 1 tbsp curry powder
- Salt to taste

Instructions

1. Combine ingredients in a saucepan.
2. Simmer 10–15 minutes.
3. Serve over rice.

Your Notes...

Creamy Coconut Chickpea Curry

Serves: 3

Ingredients

- 1 can chickpeas
- 1 can coconut milk
- 1 tbsp curry powder
- ½ tsp turmeric
- 1 tsp garlic powder
- Salt to taste

Instructions

1. Add all ingredients to a pot.
2. Simmer for **10 minutes** until thick and fragrant.
3. Serve with rice or flatbread.

Your Notes...

Tomato Chickpea Curry

Serves: 3

Ingredients

- 1 can chickpeas
- 1 can diced tomatoes
- 1 tbsp curry powder
- ½ tsp paprika
- 1 tsp garlic powder
- 1 tbsp olive oil

Instructions

1. Heat olive oil in a pot.
2. Add tomatoes and spices.
3. Stir in chickpeas.
4. Simmer **15 minutes**.

Your Notes...

Spicy Chickpea Curry

Ingredients **Serves:** 3

- 1 can chickpeas
- 1 can coconut milk
- 1 can of tomatoes
- 1 tbsp curry powder
- ½ tsp chilli flakes
- 1 tsp garlic powder

Instructions

1. Combine all ingredients in a saucepan.
2. Simmer **15 minutes**, stirring occasionally.
3. Adjust chilli to taste.

Your Notes...

Chickpea & Lentil Curry

Serves: 4

Ingredients

- 1 can chickpeas
- ½ cup dried lentils
- 1 can coconut milk
- 1 tbsp curry powder
- 4 cups water or broth
- 1 tsp garlic powder

Instructions

1. Simmer lentils in water for **15 minutes**.
2. Add chickpeas, coconut milk, and spices.
3. Cook another **10 minutes**.

Your Notes...

Chickpea Curry

Serves: 3

Ingredients

- 1 can chickpeas
- 1 can of tomatoes
- 1 tbsp curry powder
- 1 tsp garlic powder
- 1 tbsp dried parsley or dried greens
- 1 tbsp olive oil

Instructions

1. Heat olive oil in a saucepan.
2. Add tomatoes, spices, and chickpeas.
3. Stir in dried herbs.
4. Simmer **10–15 minutes**.

Your Notes...

Chickpea & Potato-Style Curry

(Using instant potatoes)

Serves: 3–4

Ingredients

- 1 can chickpeas
- 1 can of tomatoes
- 1 tbsp curry powder
- ½ cup instant mashed potato flakes
- 1½ cups water
- 1 tsp garlic powder

Instructions

1. Simmer chickpeas, tomatoes, and spices for **10 minutes**.
2. Stir in potato flakes to thicken.
3. Cook another **5 minutes**.

Your Notes...

Peanut Chickpea Curry

Serves: 3

Ingredients

- 1 can chickpeas
- 1 can coconut milk
- 2 tbsp peanut butter
- 1 tbsp curry powder
- 1 tsp garlic powder

Instructions

1. Combine all ingredients in a saucepan.
2. Stir until the peanut butter dissolves.
3. Simmer **10 minutes**.

Your Notes...

Meat-Based Meals

Canned meats are one of the most practical and reliable protein sources for a well-stocked pantry. Products such as canned chicken, canned beef, Spam, corned beef, tuna, and other preserved meats can be stored for long periods without refrigeration and are ready to use whenever needed.

Because these foods are already cooked and preserved, they can be quickly incorporated into a wide variety of meals using other pantry staples. Ingredients such as rice, pasta, dried potatoes, canned vegetables, and simple sauces make it easy to prepare filling and satisfying dishes with minimal preparation.

Canned meats are particularly useful during busy days, when fresh food is unavailable, or when cooking resources may be limited. Many of the recipes in this chapter are designed to be prepared in a single pot or skillet using simple ingredients that store well in the pantry.

These meals demonstrate how shelf-stable foods can be combined to create hearty, nourishing dishes that provide both comfort and practicality when fresh ingredients are not available.

Canned Chicken and Rice Skillet

Serves: 3–4

Ingredients

1 cup rice

1 can of canned chicken, drained

1 can of mixed vegetables

2 cups water or broth

1 tsp garlic powder

1 tbsp cooking oil

Salt and pepper to taste

Instructions

1. Heat oil in a large pan or pot.
2. Add rice and stir for 1 minute.
3. Add water or broth and bring to a simmer.
4. Stir in canned chicken and vegetables.
5. Cook until the rice is tender and the liquid is absorbed.
6. Season with garlic powder, salt, and pepper.

Your Notes...

Spam and Fried Rice

Serves: 3

Ingredients

1 cup cooked rice

1 can Spam, diced

1 cup canned vegetables

1 tbsp oil

1 tbsp soy sauce

½ tsp garlic powder

Instructions

1. Heat oil in a skillet.
2. Cook diced Spam until lightly browned.
3. Add rice and vegetables.
4. Stir in soy sauce and garlic powder.
5. Cook for several minutes until heated through.

Your Notes...

Creamy Chicken Pantry Pasta

Serves: 4

Ingredients

250 g pasta

1 can of canned chicken

1 can of evaporated milk

½ cup canned mushrooms

1 tsp garlic powder

Salt and pepper

Instructions

1. Cook pasta according to package instructions.
2. In a saucepan, combine chicken, mushrooms, and evaporated milk.
3. Add garlic powder and heat gently.
4. Stir cooked pasta into the sauce and season to taste.

Your Notes...

Corned Beef and Potato Skillet

Serves: 3–4

Ingredients

1 can corned beef

2 cups instant mashed potato flakes

2 cups water

1 can of canned corn

1 tbsp oil

½ tsp onion powder

Instructions

1. Heat oil in a skillet.
2. Add corned beef and cook until lightly browned.
3. Prepare instant mashed potatoes using water.
4. Stir potatoes and corn into the skillet with the corned beef.
5. Season with onion powder and mix well.

Your Notes...

Spam and Pasta Tomato Bowl

Serves: 3

Ingredients

250 g pasta

1 can Spam, diced

1 can diced tomatoes

1 tsp garlic powder

1 tsp dried herbs

1 tbsp olive oil

Instructions

1. Cook pasta and drain.
2. Heat olive oil in a pan and cook diced Spam until browned.
3. Add tomatoes, garlic powder, and herbs.
4. Simmer for 5–10 minutes.
5. Stir in cooked pasta and mix well.

Your Notes...

Chicken and Couscous Pantry Bowl

Serves: 3

Ingredients

1 cup couscous

1 can canned chicken

1 cup boiling water

½ cup canned vegetables

1 tbsp olive oil

Salt and pepper

Instructions

1. Place couscous in a bowl and add boiling water.
2. Cover and let sit for 5 minutes.
3. Fluff with a fork.
4. Stir in chicken, vegetables, and olive oil.
5. Season to taste.

Your Notes...

Corned Beef and Rice Stew

Serves: 4

Ingredients

1 cup rice

1 can corned beef

1 can tomatoes

3 cups water or broth

1 tsp paprika

1 tsp garlic powder

Instructions

1. Combine all ingredients in a pot.
2. Bring to a boil.
3. Reduce the heat and simmer until the rice is cooked.
4. Stir occasionally and adjust seasoning.

Your Notes...

Spam and Potato Hash

Serves: 3

Ingredients

1 can Spam, diced

2 cups instant mashed potatoes prepared

1 tbsp oil

1 tsp garlic powder

1 tsp dried herbs

Instructions

1. Heat oil in a skillet.
2. Cook Spam until browned.
3. Add prepared potatoes.
4. Season with garlic powder and herbs.
5. Stir and cook until heated through.

Your Notes...

Pantry Chicken Noodle Soup

Serves: 4

Ingredients

1 cup noodles

1 can of canned chicken

1 can of mixed vegetables

4 cups water or broth

1 tsp garlic powder

Salt and pepper

Instructions

1. Bring water or broth to a boil.
2. Add noodles and cook until tender.
3. Stir in chicken and vegetables.
4. Season and simmer for 5 minutes.

Your Notes...

Quick Spam Ramen Bowl

Serves: 2

Ingredients

2 packets of ramen noodles

1 can Spam, diced

2 cups water

½ tsp garlic powder

1 tbsp soy sauce

Instructions

1. Bring water to a boil and cook ramen noodles.
2. In a separate pan, cook Spam until browned.
3. Add Spam and soy sauce to the ramen.
4. Stir well and serve hot.

Your Notes...

Meals with Canned Fish

Canned fish is one of the most underrated ingredients in a pantry. It's inexpensive, protein-rich, shelf-stable for years, and surprisingly versatile. With just a few non-perishable ingredients, canned tuna, salmon, sardines, or mackerel can become quick meals that require little effort—sometimes no cooking at all.

Your Notes...

Mediterranean Tuna & Bean Salad

A bright, filling meal that comes together in minutes.

Ingredients

- 1 can tuna, drained
- 1 can cannellini or white beans, drained
- 2 tablespoons olive oil
- 1 tablespoon bottled lemon juice
- 1 teaspoon dried oregano
- Salt and pepper
- Optional: jarred olives

Instructions

1. Combine tuna and beans in a bowl.
2. Add olive oil, lemon juice, oregano, salt and pepper.
3. Toss gently until combined.

This dish is filling on its own or can be served on crackers.

Your Notes...

Sardine Cracker Plate

Simple, satisfying, and surprisingly elegant.

Ingredients

- 1 can of sardines in olive oil
- Crackers
- 1 tablespoon mustard
- 1 tablespoon jarred capers (optional)
- Black pepper

Instructions

1. Spread mustard on crackers.
2. Add sardines.
3. Sprinkle capers and black pepper.

Serve open-faced like small tapas.

Your Notes...

Salmon Pantry Salad

A protein-packed meal using simple staples.

Ingredients

- 1 can of salmon
- 2 tablespoons mayonnaise (shelf-stable packets or jar)
- 1 tablespoon pickle relish
- 1 teaspoon mustard
- Black pepper
- Crackers or crispbread

Instructions

1. Mix salmon, mayonnaise, relish and mustard.
2. Season with pepper.
3. Serve on crackers.

Your Notes...

Tuna Chickpea Bowl

A hearty, no-cook pantry meal.

Ingredients

- 1 can tuna
- 1 can chickpeas, drained
- 2 tablespoons olive oil
- 1 teaspoon garlic powder
- 1 teaspoon dried parsley
- Salt and pepper

Instructions

1. Combine all ingredients in a bowl.
2. Mix well and adjust seasoning.

This dish keeps well for several hours and works great for packed lunches.

Your Notes...

Creamy Tuna Pasta

Comfort food made entirely from shelf staples.

Ingredients

- 200 g dried pasta
- 1 can of tuna
- 1 cup powdered milk prepared as milk
- 1 tablespoon butter powder or oil
- 1 teaspoon garlic powder
- Salt and pepper

Instructions

1. Cook pasta according to package instructions.
2. Drain and return to pot.
3. Stir in tuna, prepared powdered milk, butter powder and garlic powder.
4. Season with salt and pepper.

Your Notes...

Sardine Tomato Rice

Simple, rich and satisfying.

Ingredients

- 1 cup instant rice
- 1 can of sardines in tomato sauce (or sardines plus canned tomatoes)
- 1 teaspoon garlic powder
- ½ teaspoon chilli flakes (optional)

Instructions

1. Prepare instant rice according to directions.
2. Stir in sardines and sauce.
3. Add garlic powder and chilli flakes.

Heat until warmed through.

Your Notes...

Mackerel Pantry Hash

A quick skillet meal with bold flavour.

Ingredients

- 1 can mackerel
- 1 cup canned potatoes, drained
- 1 tablespoon oil
- 1 teaspoon paprika
- ½ teaspoon onion powder
- Salt and pepper

Instructions

1. Heat oil in a skillet.
2. Add potatoes and cook until lightly crisp.
3. Stir in mackerel and spices.
4. Cook 2–3 minutes until heated.

Your Notes...

The Kids Only Want Nuggets

In an ideal world, children would calmly eat lentil stew and canned vegetables without complaint. In reality, many of us are raising children who have a very clear idea of what food should look like, taste like, and feel like.

For a lot of families, that means chicken nuggets, crackers, pasta, and anything that comes in a bright box with a cartoon character on the front.

When life runs smoothly, this is mostly an inconvenience. When times are difficult—when supply chains falter, money is tight, or you're relying heavily on what is already in the pantry—it can feel like a disaster.

Parents often worry: *What if the only food I have isn't what my child will eat?*

The truth is that most "kid foods" can actually be recreated from basic pantry staples. They may not come in a freezer bag shaped like dinosaurs, but they can taste familiar enough to keep small critics satisfied.

The key is understanding **why kids like those foods**.

Children tend to prefer foods that are:

- Mild in flavour
- Crispy or crunchy
- Uniform in texture
- Easy to dip
- Familiar in shape

With a few pantry basics—flour, canned chicken, beans, oats, breadcrumbs, powdered milk, and canned vegetables—you can recreate many of the foods kids already love.

Below are a few simple recipes designed specifically with **picky eaters in mind**.

Your Notes...

Pantry "Chicken" Nuggets

When kids ask for nuggets, they're usually craving the crispy outside and soft middle. Canned chicken works surprisingly well for this.

Pantry ingredients

- 1 can chicken, drained
- ½ cup breadcrumbs or crushed crackers
- 1 egg (or 2 tbsp powdered egg mixed with water)
- 2 tbsp flour
- ½ tsp salt
- ½ tsp garlic powder (optional)
- Oil for frying

Instructions

1. In a bowl, mash the canned chicken until finely shredded.
2. Mix in egg, flour, salt, and half the breadcrumbs.
3. Form small nugget shapes with your hands.
4. Roll nuggets in the remaining breadcrumbs.
5. Pan-fry in a shallow layer of oil until golden on both sides.

Serve with tomato sauce, honey mustard, or even canned tomato sauce for dipping.

Crispy Bean Nuggets (Hidden Protein)

This version works well when meat is limited. The flavour is mild enough that many kids won't even realise they're eating beans.

Ingredients

- 1 cup canned white beans or chickpeas, mashed
- ½ cup breadcrumbs
- 2 tbsp flour
- 1 egg or powdered egg substitute
- ¼ tsp salt
- ½ tsp onion powder (optional)

Instructions

1. Mash beans until smooth.
2. Mix with egg, flour, salt, and half the breadcrumbs.
3. Shape into nuggets or small patties.
4. Coat in remaining breadcrumbs.
5. Pan-fry until crisp and golden.

Serve exactly the same way as chicken nuggets.

The dipping sauce is often what convinces kids to eat them.

Pantry Mac & Cheese

Most children will eat pasta even when they refuse everything else. With powdered milk and basic pantry ingredients, you can create a simple cheese sauce.

Ingredients

- 2 cups dry macaroni or small pasta
- 2 tbsp butter or oil
- 2 tbsp flour
- 1 cup water
- ¼ cup powdered milk
- ½–¾ cup shredded cheese (or powdered cheese if available)
- Salt to taste

Instructions

1. Cook pasta according to package instructions.
2. In a pot, melt butter and stir in flour to make a paste.
3. Slowly add water and powdered milk while whisking.
4. Stir until thickened.
5. Add cheese and stir until melted.
6. Mix with cooked pasta.

For picky eaters, keep the seasoning simple.

Crispy Pantry Pizza Toast

Kids love pizza flavours, and canned or shelf-stable ingredients work perfectly.

Ingredients

- Bread or flatbread
- Tomato paste or canned tomato sauce
- Dried Italian seasoning
- Shelf-stable pepperoni, canned chicken, or beans
- Shredded cheese (or powdered cheese)

Instructions

1. Spread tomato sauce on bread.
2. Sprinkle seasoning.
3. Add toppings and cheese.
4. Bake or cook in a covered pan until the cheese melts.

This recipe works even in a skillet if an oven isn't available.

Your Notes...

No-Bake Pantry Cookie Bites

When routines change, children often crave sweets even more than usual. These simple cookie bites require no oven.

Ingredients

- 1 cup oats
- ½ cup peanut butter (or other nut/seed butter)
- ¼ cup honey or sugar syrup
- 2 tbsp powdered milk (optional)
- 2 tbsp cocoa powder or chocolate chips

Instructions

1. Mix everything in a bowl.
2. Roll into small balls.
3. Chill if possible, or eat as is.

These provide quick energy and feel like a treat during stressful times.

Your Notes...

No-Cook Pantry Meals

Sometimes cooking simply isn't possible. Power outages, camping trips, travel, emergencies, or extreme heat can make using a stove or oven difficult or unsafe. During these times, having a pantry stocked with shelf-stable foods allows you to prepare nourishing meals without needing to cook.

Many foods are ready to eat straight from the pantry, including canned beans, fish, vegetables, grains, spreads, and dried fruits. With a little creativity, these ingredients can be combined to create meals that are filling, balanced, and surprisingly satisfying.

The recipes in this chapter require **no cooking at all**. They rely on simple preparation—opening, mixing, assembling, or soaking ingredients that soften on their own. These meals are designed to be practical and convenient while still providing energy and nutrition.

Whether you are preparing for emergencies, packing food for a camping trip, or simply need a quick meal without turning on the stove, these no-cook recipes show how versatile pantry foods can be.

Tuna & White Bean Salad

Serves: 2

Mix together:

- 1 can of tuna
- 1 can white beans, drained
- 1 tbsp olive oil
- 1 tbsp vinegar
- Salt and pepper

Serve with crackers.

Your Notes...

Chickpea Salad Bowl

Serves: 2

Mix:

- 1 can chickpeas
- 1 tbsp olive oil
- ½ tsp paprika
- 1 tbsp lemon juice or vinegar
- Salt and pepper

Sardine Crackers

Serves: 1

Top whole grain crackers with:

- Canned sardines
- A drizzle of olive oil
- Salt, Black pepper

Your Notes...

Peanut Butter Energy Wrap

Serves: 1

Spread on flatbread or tortilla:

- 2 tbsp peanut butter
- Honey
- Dried fruit

Roll and eat.

Pantry Pasta Salad

Serves: 2

Combine:

- Cooked shelf-stable pasta pouch or pre-cooked pasta
- 1 can of tuna
- ½ cup canned corn
- Olive oil
- Garlic powder

Your Notes...

Bean & Corn Salad

Serves: 2

Mix:

- 1 can black beans
- 1 can of corn
- 1 tbsp olive oil
- Chilli powder
- Salt and pepper

Crackers with Bean Spread

Serves: 1–2

Mash:

- 1 can chickpeas
- 1 tbsp olive oil
- Garlic powder

Spread on crackers.

Your Notes...

Couscous Soak Bowl

Serves: 2

Combine in a bowl:

- 1 cup couscous
- 1 cup hot tap water
- ½ cup canned vegetables

Let it sit for 10 minutes until soft.

Tuna Rice Salad

Serves: 2

Mix:

- Pre-cooked rice pouch
- 1 can of tuna
- Olive oil
- Pepper

Your Notes...

Peanut Butter Granola Bowl

Serves: 1

Combine:

- Granola
- Peanut butter
- Dried fruit
- Shelf-stable milk

Hummus

Ingredients

- 1 can chickpeas (400g), drained
- 2–3 tbsp olive oil
- 1–2 tbsp lemon juice (bottled is fine)
- 1 small garlic clove **or** ½ tsp garlic powder
- ½ tsp salt (adjust to taste)
- ½ tsp ground cumin (optional but nice)
- 2–4 tbsp water or liquid from the chickpea can

Method

1. Drain chickpeas (reserve a little of the liquid).
2. Mash or blend chickpeas and other ingredients
3. Blend until smooth.
4. Add water or chickpea liquid until creamy.
5. Taste and adjust salt/lemon.
6. Drizzle with olive oil and sprinkle paprika if you like.

No blender?
Mash chickpeas very well with a fork or potato masher and stir in the other ingredients.

Spread mashed beans on a homemade tortilla with olive oil and spices, then roll up.

Savoury Pantry Pastries

Savoury pastries have long been a practical and satisfying way to turn simple ingredients into a filling meal. A basic pastry dough made from flour, fat, and water can be transformed into pies, rolls, turnovers, and hand-held pastries that are both comforting and convenient.

Even when fresh ingredients are limited, a well-stocked pantry can provide everything needed to create delicious savoury pastries. Canned beans, lentils, tuna, chicken, vegetables, and dried herbs make excellent fillings, while simple pantry doughs provide the perfect golden crust.

Many of these pastries are easy to prepare and can be baked in a standard oven, cooked in a skillet, or even prepared over a campfire or barbecue. They are ideal for lunches, dinners, or portable meals when cooking facilities are limited.

This chapter offers simple, practical recipes that transform pantry staples into hearty pastries that bring warmth and comfort to the table.

Basic Pantry Pastry Dough

Makes: enough for one pie or 6 small pastries

Ingredients

- 2 cups flour
- ½ tsp salt
- ½ cup vegetable oil or shortening
- ¼–½ cup cold water

Instructions

1. Mix flour and salt in a bowl.
2. Stir in oil until crumbly.
3. Add water gradually until the dough forms.
4. Roll out for pies or pastries.

Your Notes...

Tuna & Tomato Hand Pies

Serves: 4

Ingredients

- Pantry pastry dough
- 1 can tuna
- ½ cup canned diced tomatoes (drained)
- ½ tsp garlic powder
- Salt and pepper

Instructions

1. Mix tuna, tomatoes, and spices.
2. Roll the dough and cut into circles.
3. Place filling on half the circle and fold over.
4. Bake **20–25 minutes at 180°C / 350°F**.

Your Notes...

Chickpea Curry Pastry Pockets

Serves: 4

Ingredients

- Pantry pastry dough
- 1 cup chickpea curry (from pantry curry recipes)

Instructions

1. Spoon curry into pastry circles.
2. Fold into triangles.
3. Bake **20 minutes at 180°C / 350°F**.

Your Notes...

Lentil & Herb Savoury Pie

Serves: 4–6

Ingredients

- Pantry pastry dough
- 1 cup cooked lentils
- 1 tsp garlic powder
- 1tbs onion powder
- salt
- 1 tsp or more dried herbs
- ½ cup canned vegetables

Instructions

1. Mix filling ingredients.
2. Line a pie dish with pastry.
3. Add filling and top with pastry lid.
4. Bake **30 minutes at 180°C / 350°F**.

Your Notes...

Bean & Corn Empanadas

Serves: 4

Ingredients

- Pantry pastry dough
- 1 cup black beans
- ½ cup canned corn
- ½ tsp cumin
- ½ tsp paprika

Instructions

1. Mix beans, corn, and spices.
2. Fill pastry circles and fold over.
3. Bake **20–25 minutes**.

Your Notes...

Savoury Crackers

Makes: about 20 crackers

Ingredients

- 1 cup flour
- ½ tsp salt
- 2 tbsp oil
- ¼ cup water
- ½ tsp dried herbs

Instructions

1. Mix ingredients int dough.
2. Roll thin and cut into squares.
3. Bake **12–15 minutes at 180°C / 350°F**.

Your Notes...

Pantry Pot Pie

Serves: 4

Ingredients

- Pastry dough
- 1 can chicken or chickpeas
- 1 cup canned vegetables
- 1 cup evaporated milk
- 1 tsp garlic powder

Instructions

1. Mix filling ingredients and place in a baking dish.
2. Cover with pastry.
3. Bake **30 minutes at 180°C / 350°F**.

Your Notes...

Savoury Onion-Style Turnovers

(Using dried onion flakes)

Serves: 4

Ingredients

- Pastry dough
- 2 tbsp dried onion flakes
- 1 tsp garlic powder
- ½ cup canned mushrooms
- 1 tbsp oil

Instructions

1. Mix filling ingredients.
2. Fill pastry circles and seal edges.
3. Bake **20 minutes**.

Your Notes...

Chickpea & Tomato Pie

Serves: 4

Ingredients

- Pastry dough
- 1 can chickpeas
- 1 can diced tomatoes (drained)
- 1 tsp curry powder

Instructions

1. Combine filling ingredients.
2. Place in a pastry-lined dish.
3. Add pastry lid and bake **30 minutes**.

Your Notes...

Savoury Pizza Pastry Squares

Serves: 4

Ingredients

- Pastry dough
- ½ cup canned tomatoes
- 1 tsp garlic powder
- 1 tsp dried herbs
- ½ cup canned vegetables

Instructions

1. Roll the dough into a rectangle.
2. Spread tomatoes and vegetables on top.
3. Sprinkle herbs.
4. Bake **20 minutes at 180°C / 350°F**.

Your Notes...

Sweet Pantry Pastries

Sweet pastries are a comforting treat that can be enjoyed at any time of the day. While many pastries traditionally rely on fresh ingredients, it is still possible to create delicious baked sweets using simple pantry staples.

Basic ingredients such as flour, sugar, oil, powdered milk, dried fruit, and canned fruit can be used to create a wide variety of pastries, from turnovers and tarts to rolls and sweet pies. With just a few ingredients and a simple dough, these pantry pastries can be prepared easily and enjoyed warm from the oven.

These recipes are designed to be practical and flexible, using ingredients that store well and are commonly found in the pantry. Whether you are baking for a family dessert, a special occasion, or simply a comforting treat, these sweet pastries prove that delicious baking is possible even when fresh ingredients are limited.

Basic Sweet Pastry Dough

Makes: 1 pie or 6 small pastries

Ingredients

- 2 cups flour
- ¼ cup sugar
- ½ tsp salt
- ½ cup vegetable oil or shortening
- ¼–½ cup cold water

Instructions

1. Mix flour, sugar, and salt.
2. Stir in oil until crumbly.
3. Add water gradually until the dough forms.
4. Roll out for pastries or pies.

Your Notes...

Canned Fruit Turnovers

Serves: 4

Ingredients

- Sweet pastry dough
- 1 cup canned fruit (drained)
- 1 tbsp sugar
- ½ tsp cinnamon

Instructions

1. Mix fruit, sugar, and cinnamon.
2. Place filling on pastry circles.
3. Fold over and seal edges.
4. Bake **20–25 minutes at 180°C / 350°F**.

Your Notes...

Apple Cinnamon Hand Pies

Serves: 4

Ingredients

- Sweet pastry dough
- 1 cup canned apples or applesauce
- 1 tbsp sugar
- ½ tsp cinnamon

Instructions

1. Place apple filling onto pastry circles.
2. Fold and seal.
3. Bake at **180 °C for 20 minutes** until golden.

Your Notes...

Chocolate Pastry Pockets

Serves: 4

Ingredients

- Sweet pastry dough
- ½ cup chocolate chips
- 1 tbsp sugar

Instructions

1. Place chocolate chips in pastry circles.
2. Fold and seal edges.
3. Bake at **180 °C** for **18–20 minutes**.

Your Notes...

Peanut Butter Pastry Rolls

Serves: 4

Ingredients

- Sweet pastry dough
- ½ cup peanut butter
- 2 tbsp honey or sugar

Instructions

1. Spread peanut butter over the rolled pastry.
2. Drizzle honey.
3. Roll the dough and slice into spirals.
4. Bake at **170 °C** for **20 minutes**.

Your notes...

Raisin Cinnamon Pastry Swirls

Serves: 6

Ingredients

- Sweet pastry dough
- ½ cup raisins
- 2 tbsp sugar
- 1 tsp cinnamon

Instructions

1. Spread raisins, sugar, and cinnamon over the pastry.
2. Roll dough into a log.
3. Slice and bake at **180 °C** for **20 minutes**.

Your notes....

Honey Nut Pastry Bites

Serves: 6

Ingredients

- Sweet pastry dough
- ½ cup chopped nuts
- 3 tbsp honey

Instructions

1. Fill pastry squares with nuts and honey.
2. Fold into small parcels.
3. Bake at **180 °C for 18–20 minutes**.

Your Notes...

Chocolate Oat Pastry Tart

Serves: 6

Ingredients

- Sweet pastry dough
- ½ cup oats
- 2 tbsp cocoa powder
- 3 tbsp honey

Instructions

1. Mix oats, cocoa, and honey.
2. Spread into a pastry-lined tart dish.
3. Bake at **180 °C for 25 minutes**.

Your Notes...

Jam Pastry Squares

Serves: 6

Ingredients

- Sweet pastry dough
- ½ cup jam or fruit spread

Instructions

1. Press pastry into a baking dish.
2. Spread jam on top.
3. Bake at **180 °C for 20–25 minutes**.
4. Cut into squares.

Your Notes...

Coconut Sweet Pastry Tart

Serves: 6

Ingredients

- Sweet pastry dough
- ½ cup shredded coconut
- 3 tbsp sugar
- ½ cup powdered milk mixture

Instructions

1. Mix coconut, sugar, and milk mixture.
2. Pour into pastry shell.
3. Bake at **175 °C** for **25 minutes**.

Your Notes…

Pantry Sweet Treats

A sweet treat can bring comfort at the end of a long day or add a little celebration to an ordinary moment. Even when fresh ingredients are limited, a well-stocked pantry can provide everything needed to create simple and satisfying desserts.

Many classic sweets rely on ingredients that store well for long periods—flour, oats, sugar, honey, cocoa powder, dried fruit, canned fruit, peanut butter, coconut, nuts, and shelf-stable milk. With these pantry staples, it is possible to prepare a wide variety of desserts, from cakes and pastries to biscuits, candies, and quick no-bake treats.

The recipes in this section are designed to be practical and approachable, using ingredients that are easy to keep on hand. Some recipes are baked, while others can be mixed together quickly for a sweet snack or dessert with very little preparation.

Whether you are baking a simple cake, preparing a sweet pastry, or making homemade candies, these recipes show how versatile pantry ingredients can be. Even with the most basic supplies, it is still possible to create delicious treats that bring warmth, comfort, and a little sweetness to the table.

Oatmeal Cookie Bars

These simple bars are made using basic pantry ingredients and are suitable as a snack or dessert.

Serves: 8

Ingredients

- 1 cup rolled oats.
- 1 cup plain flour.
- ½ cup sugar.
- ⅓ cup vegetable oil.
- ½ cup raisins.
- ½ cup water.

Instructions

1. Preheat the oven to **170°C** and lightly grease or line a small baking dish.
2. In a bowl, combine the **rolled oats, flour, sugar, and raisins**.
3. Add the **oil and water** and mix until well combined.
4. Press the mixture evenly into the prepared dish.
5. Bake for **20 minutes** or until lightly golden.
6. Allow to cool before cutting into bars.

Simple Jam Crumble Bars

Serves: 6–8 bars

Ingredients

- 1 cup all-purpose flour
- ½ cup rolled oats
- ½ cup sugar (white or brown sugar)
- ½ cup butter or margarine, softened
- ½–¾ cup fruit jam or preserves (any flavour)
- ½ teaspoon vanilla extract (optional)
- A pinch of salt

Instructions

1. Preheat the oven to **180°C / 350°F**.
2. Lightly grease, or line a small baking dish
3. In a mixing bowl, combine the flour, oats, sugar, and salt.
4. Add the softened butter and mix until the ingredients form a crumbly dough.
5. Press about **two-thirds of the mixture** evenly into the bottom of the prepared baking dish to form the base.
6. Spread the jam evenly over the dough layer.
7. Sprinkle the remaining crumb mixture over the jam to create the crumble topping.
8. Bake for **20–25 minutes**, or until the top is lightly golden.

Simple Pantry Vanilla Cake

Serves: 8

Ingredients

- 1½ cups flour
- ¾ cup sugar
- 1 tsp baking powder
- ½ tsp salt
- ½ cup powdered milk mixture
- ¼ cup oil
- 1 tsp vanilla (optional)

Instructions

1. Preheat oven to **180°C / 350°F**.
2. Mix flour, sugar, baking powder, and salt.
3. Stir in milk mixture, oil, and vanilla.
4. Pour into a greased pan.
5. Bake **25–30 minutes**.

Your Notes...

Peanut Butter Oat Bars

Serves: 8

Ingredients

- 2 cups oats
- ½ cup peanut butter
- ⅓ cup honey
- ¼ cup chocolate chips (optional)

Instructions

1. Mix all ingredients together.
2. Press into a lined pan.
3. Chill for 1 hour before cutting.

Your Notes....

Chocolate Pantry Cake

Serves: 8

Ingredients

- 1½ cups flour
- ¾ cup sugar
- ¼ cup cocoa powder
- 1 tsp baking powder
- ½ cup powdered milk mixture
- ¼ cup oil

Instructions

1. Mix dry ingredients.
2. Add milk mixture and oil.
3. Pour into the cake pan.
4. Bake **25–30 minutes at 180°C / 350°F**.

Your Notes...

Pantry Caramel Cake

Serves: 8

Ingredients

- 1½ cups flour
- ¾ cup brown sugar
- 1 tsp baking powder
- ½ cup powdered milk mixture
- ¼ cup oil

Instructions

1. Mix dry ingredients.
2. Stir in milk mixture and oil.
3. Bake **25–30 minutes at 180°C / 350°F**.

Your Notes...

Cinnamon Tea Cake

Serves: 8

Ingredients

- 1½ cups flour
- ½ cup sugar
- 1 tsp baking powder
- 1 tsp cinnamon
- ½ cup powdered milk mixture
- ¼ cup oil

Instructions

1. Mix dry ingredients.
2. Stir in milk mixture and oil.
3. Bake **25 minutes at 180°C / 350°F**.

Your Notes...

Pantry Fruit Cake

Serves: 8

Ingredients

- 1½ cups flour
- ½ cup sugar
- 1 tsp baking powder
- 1 cup dried fruit
- ½ cup powdered milk mixture
- ¼ cup oil
- ½ tsp cinnamon

Instructions

1. Mix dry ingredients and dried fruit.
2. Add milk mixture and oil.
3. Bake **30 minutes at 180°C / 350°F**.

Your Notes...

No-Bake Cheesecake Style Dessert

Serves: 6

Ingredients

- 1 cup crushed crackers or biscuits
- 3 tbsp melted butter or oil
- 1 cup powdered milk mixture (thick)
- 3 tbsp lemon juice
- 3 tbsp honey or sugar

Instructions

1. Mix crushed crackers with butter and press into the dish.
2. Mix milk mixture, lemon juice, and honey until thick and creamy.
3. Spread over the crust.
4. Chill for 1–2 hours.

Your Notes...

Simple Rice Pudding

Serves: 3

Ingredients

- 1 cup cooked rice
- 1 cup evaporated milk
- 2 tbsp sugar
- ¼ tsp cinnamon
- ¼ cup raisins

Instructions

1. Combine all ingredients in a saucepan.
2. Simmer gently for 10 minutes.

Your Notes...

Honey Granola Clusters

Serves: 4

Ingredients

- 2 cups rolled oats
- ⅓ cup honey
- ¼ cup chopped nuts (almonds, peanuts, or walnuts)
- 1 tablespoon cooking oil (vegetable, coconut, or olive oil)
- A pinch of salt

Instructions

1. Preheat the oven to **180°C / 350°F**.
2. Line a baking tray with baking paper or lightly grease it.
3. Combine the oats, chopped nuts, and salt.
4. Add the honey and oil,Stir.
5. If using optional ingredients such as seeds or coconut, mix them in now.
6. Spread the mixture evenly on the prepared baking tray.
7. Bake for **about 12–15 minutes**, stirring once halfway through, until the granola is lightly golden.
8. Remove from the oven and allow it to cool completely. As it cools, the granola will form small clusters.
9. Stir in dried fruit or chocolate chips after the granola has cooled.

No-Bake Chocolate Oat Balls

Serves: About 12 balls

Ingredients

- 1 cup rolled oats
- 2 tablespoons cocoa powder
- ½ cup peanut butter
- ⅓ cup honey or golden syrup
- ½ teaspoon vanilla extract (optional)
- A pinch of salt

Instructions

1. In a medium bowl, combine the oats, cocoa powder, and salt.
2. Add the peanut butter and honey (or golden syrup).
3. Stir well until the mixture becomes thick and evenly combined.
4. Mix in any optional ingredients such as coconut, nuts, or dried fruit.
5. Using your hands or a spoon, roll the mixture into small balls about the size of a tablespoon.
6. Place the balls on a plate or tray lined with baking paper.
7. Refrigerate for **about 30 minutes** to allow them to firm up.
8. Once chilled, store them in an airtight container.

Chocolate Cheesecake Substitute

Serves: 6

Ingredients

- 1 cup crushed biscuits or crackers
- 3 tbsp butter or oil
- 1 cup thick powdered milk mixture
- 2 tbsp cocoa powder
- 3 tbsp honey

Instructions

1. Press biscuit mixture into the dish for the crust.
2. Mix milk mixture, cocoa, and honey.
3. Spread over the crust and chill.

Your Notes...

Coconut Oat Cookies

These simple cookies use basic pantry ingredients and are quick to prepare.

Serves: 12

Ingredients

• 1 cup rolled oats.
• ½ cup desiccated coconut.
• ½ cup sugar.
• ⅓ cup vegetable oil.
• ½ cup prepared powdered milk • 1 cup plain flour.
• 1 teaspoon baking powder.

Method

1. Preheat the oven to **180°C** and line a baking tray with baking paper.
2. In a bowl, combine the rolled oats, coconut, sugar, flour, and baking powder.
3. Add the oil and milk and mix until a soft dough forms.
4. Roll into small balls. Flatten slightly.
5. Bake for **15 minutes** or until lightly golden.
6. Allow the cookies to cool on the tray before transferring to a wire rack.

No-Bake Peanut Butter Cookies

These quick cookies require no baking and use simple pantry ingredients.

Serves: 12

Ingredients

- 1 cup peanut butter.
- ½ cup sugar.
- 1 cup rolled oats.

Method

1. In a bowl, combine the **peanut butter and sugar** and mix until smooth.
2. Stir in the **rolled oats** until well combined.
3. Shape the mixture into small cookies or balls and place them on a tray or plate.
4. Refrigerate for **30 minutes** or until firm.

Your Notes...

Oatmeal Pantry Biscuits (Cookies)

Makes: 12

Ingredients

- 1 cup oats
- ¾ cup flour
- ½ cup sugar
- ½ tsp baking soda
- ¼ cup oil
- ¼ cup powdered milk mixture
- ½ cup raisins

Instructions

1. Mix all ingredients.
2. Drop spoonfuls onto the baking tray.
3. Bake **12–15 minutes at 180°C / 350°F**.

Your Notes...

Chocolate Crackle Biscuits

Makes: 12

Ingredients

- 1 cup oats or puffed rice cereal
- ¼ cup cocoa powder
- ½ cup peanut butter
- ⅓ cup honey

Instructions

1. Mix all ingredients.
2. Shape into small biscuits or clusters.
3. Chill until firm.

Your Notes...

Peanut Butter Fudge

Ingredients

•1 cup peanut butter.

•½ cup honey.

•1 cup powdered milk.

Method

1. In a small saucepan, gently heat the peanut butter and honey over low heat until melted and smooth.
2. Remove from heat and stir in the powdered milk until well combined and thick.
3. Press the mixture evenly into a small lined dish.
4. Refrigerate for 1–2 hours or until firm.
5. Cut into 12 squares to serve.

Your Notes...

Sweet Couscous Dessert

Serves: 2

Ingredients

- ½ cup couscous.
- ½ cup hot water.
- 1–2 tablespoons honey.
- 2 tablespoons raisins.
- ½ teaspoon ground cinnamon.

Method

1. Place the **couscous** in a bowl and pour over the **hot water**.
2. Cover and allow it to stand for **5 minutes** until the water is absorbed.
3. Fluff the couscous with a fork.
4. Stir in the **honey, raisins, and cinnamon** until well combined.
5. Serve warm.

Cinnamon Rice Dessert

Serves: 2

Ingredients

- 1 cup cooked rice.
- 1 cup shelf-stable milk or prepared powdered milk.
- 2 tablespoons sugar.
- ½ teaspoon ground cinnamon.

Method

1. Place the **cooked rice** in a small saucepan.
2. Add the **milk, sugar, and cinnamon**.
3. Heat gently over low heat, stirring occasionally, until warmed through and slightly creamy.
4. Serve warm.

Pantry Apple Dessert

Warm canned apples with cinnamon and sugar.

Your Notes...

Sweet Trail Mix Treat

Mix dried fruit, nuts, chocolate chips, and coconut flakes.

Ingredients

- 1 cup peanut butter
- ½ cup sugar
- ½ cup flour
- 2 tbsp powdered milk mixture

Instructions

1. Mix all ingredients.
2. Roll into small balls and flatten.
3. Bake **10–12 minutes at 180°C / 350°F**.

Your Notes...

Pantry Caramel Sauce

This caramel sauce can be made using shelf-stable pantry ingredients and is suitable for drizzling over desserts, fruit, or pancakes.

Serves: 6

Ingredients

- 1 cup brown sugar.
- 2 tablespoons vegetable oil or coconut oil.
- ½ cup prepared powdered milk.
- 1 teaspoon vanilla extract (optional).
- Pinch of salt (optional).

Method

1. Place the brown sugar and oil in a small saucepan over medium heat.
2. Stir until the sugar begins to dissolve and the mixture becomes smooth.
3. Gradually add the prepared powdered milk, stirring constantly to combine.
4. Bring the mixture to a gentle simmer and cook for 3–5 minutes, stirring frequently, until slightly thickened.
5. Remove from heat and stir in the vanilla and salt if using.
6. Allow the sauce to cool slightly before serving.

Pantry Chocolate Sauce

This chocolate sauce can be made using simple non-perishable pantry ingredients and is suitable for desserts, cakes and pancakes.

Serves: 6

Ingredients

- ½ cup cocoa powder.
- 1 cup sugar.
- 1 cup prepared powdered milk.
- 1 teaspoon vanilla extract (optional).
- Pinch of salt (optional).

Method

1. In a small saucepan, combine the cocoa powder and sugar.
2. Stir in the prepared powdered milk until the mixture is smooth.
3. Place the saucepan over medium heat and stir continuously.
4. Bring the mixture to a gentle simmer and cook for 3–5 minutes, stirring until the sauce thickens.
5. Remove from heat and stir in the vanilla and salt if using.
6. Allow the sauce to cool slightly before serving.

Lollies and Candies

Sweet treats have always been a simple way to brighten a day. Even with only basic pantry ingredients, it is possible to create a wide variety of delicious candies and lollies at home.

Many traditional sweets rely on ingredients that store well for long periods, such as sugar, honey, cocoa powder, peanut butter, oats, dried fruit, and nuts. With just a few of these pantry staples, you can make chewy, crunchy, or chocolatey treats without needing fresh dairy or specialty ingredients.

The recipes in this section are designed to be easy to prepare and require only simple equipment. Some are cooked on the stovetop, while others are quick, no-bake sweets that can be mixed together and chilled.

These homemade lollies and candies are perfect for sharing, gifting, or simply enjoying as a small treat alongside your pantry meals.

Honey Peanut Butter Fudge

Makes: about 12 pieces

Ingredients

- 1 cup peanut butter
- ⅓ cup honey
- ½ cup powdered milk

Instructions

1. Warm peanut butter and honey together in a saucepan.
2. Stir in powdered milk until thick.
3. Press into a lined dish.
4. Chill until firm and cut into squares.

Your Notes...

Chocolate Oat Fudge

Makes: 12 squares

Ingredients

- 1 cup oats
- ½ cup peanut butter
- ¼ cup cocoa powder
- ⅓ cup honey

Instructions

1. Mix all ingredients together in a bowl.
2. Press into a small pan.
3. Refrigerate until firm and cut into squares.

Your Notes...

Coconut Honey Balls

Makes: 12

Ingredients

- 1 cup shredded coconut
- 3 tbsp honey
- 2 tbsp powdered milk
- 1 tbsp coconut oil (optional)

Instructions

1. Mix ingredients until sticky.
2. Roll into small balls.
3. Chill before serving.

Your Notes...

Honey Sesame Crunch

Makes: 10 pieces

Ingredients

- 1 cup sesame seeds
- ⅓ cup honey
- 2 tbsp sugar

Instructions

1. Heat honey and sugar in a saucepan.
2. Stir in sesame seeds.
3. Spread mixture thinly onto baking paper.
4. Cool and break into pieces.

Your Notes...

Peanut Butter Candy Balls

Makes: 12

Ingredients

- ½ cup peanut butter
- ½ cup powdered sugar
- 2 tbsp powdered milk

Instructions

1. Mix ingredients until a firm dough forms.
2. Roll into balls.
3. Chill until set.

Your Notes...

Chocolate Substitute

Ingredients

- ½ cup cocoa powder.
- ¼ cup coconut oil or vegetable oil.
- ¼ cup honey, golden syrup, or sugar.

Method

1. Gently warm the coconut oil until melted.
2. Stir in the cocoa powder and sweetener until smooth.
3. Mix well until a thick chocolate mixture forms.
4. Use immediately in recipes or pour into a lined dish and chill until firm.

Uses

This mixture can be used for:

- Coating snacks or cereal treats.
- Making simple chocolate bars or lollies.
- Drizzling over desserts.

Your Notes...

Chocolate Rice Candy

Makes: 12 pieces

Ingredients

- 1 cup puffed rice cereal
- ½ cup chocolate sauce
- 2 tbsp peanut butter

Instructions

1. Mix cereal with chocolate and peanut butter.
2. Press into a small tray.
3. Chill and cut into squares.

Your Notes...

Cinnamon Sugar Almonds

Serves: 4

Ingredients

- 1 cup almonds or mixed nuts
- 2 tbsp sugar
- ½ tsp cinnamon
- 1 tbsp honey

Instructions

1. Heat the honey in a pan.
2. Stir in nuts, sugar, and cinnamon.
3. Cook briefly until coated.
4. Cool before serving.

Your Notes...

No-Bake Chocolate Coconut Bars

Makes: 12 bars

Ingredients

- 1 cup oats
- ½ cup shredded coconut
- ¼ cup cocoa powder
- ⅓ cup honey

Instructions

1. Mix ingredients together.
2. Press into a pan.
3. Chill until firm.

Your Notes...

Toffee

Ingredients

- 1 cup brown sugar.
- ¼ cup water.
- 2 tablespoons of prepared Butter powder.
- 1 tablespoon golden syrup or honey.

Method

1. Place the brown sugar, water, butter, and golden syrup in a small saucepan.
2. Stir over low heat until the sugar has dissolved.
3. Increase the heat slightly and allow the mixture to simmer without stirring for 5–8 minutes, or until it thickens and turns a deeper golden colour.
4. Carefully pour the mixture into a lightly greased or lined dish.
5. Allow it to cool and harden completely before breaking into pieces.

Your Notes...

Honey Nut Brittle

Makes: 12 pieces

Ingredients

- 1 cup nuts
- ½ cup sugar
- ¼ cup honey

Instructions

1. Heat sugar and honey until bubbling.
2. Stir in nuts.
3. Spread onto baking paper.
4. Cool and break into pieces.

Your Notes...

Peanut Butter Chocolate Bites

Ingredients

- ½ cup cocoa powder.
- ½ cup peanut butter.
- ½ cup honey or golden syrup.
- ½ cup powdered milk.

Method

1. In a bowl, mix the peanut butter and honey until smooth.
2. Stir in the cocoa powder and powdered milk until a thick mixture forms.
3. Roll the mixture into small balls.
4. Place on a tray and refrigerate for 30 minutes until firm.

Your Notes...

Chocolate Fudge Squares

Ingredients

- ½ cup cocoa powder.
- ½ cup honey or golden syrup.
- 1 cup powdered milk.

Method

1. In a small saucepan, gently heat the honey until warm.
2. Stir in the cocoa powder and powdered milk until a thick mixture forms.
3. Press the mixture into a lined dish.
4. Refrigerate for 1–2 hours until firm.
5. Cut into small squares.

Your Notes...

Coconut Chocolate Lollies

Ingredients

- 1 cup desiccated coconut.
- 2 tablespoons cocoa powder.
- ¼ cup honey or golden syrup.
- 2 tablespoons coconut oil.

Method

1. In a bowl, combine the coconut and cocoa powder.
2. Add the honey and coconut oil and mix until the mixture holds together.
3. Press into small moulds or roll into bite-sized balls.
4. Chill in the refrigerator for 30 minutes until firm.

Your Notes...

Peanut Butter Chocolate Cups (Pantry Version)

Makes: 10

Ingredients

- ½ cup peanut butter.
- ¼ cup cocoa powder.
- ¼ cup coconut oil or vegetable oil.
- ¼ cup sugar or honey.

Instructions

1. In a small saucepan, gently warm the oil, cocoa powder, and sugar, stirring until smooth.
2. Spoon a small amount of the chocolate mixture into the bottom of small paper cups.
3. Add a small spoonful of peanut butter to each cup.
4. Cover with more of the chocolate mixture.
5. Refrigerate until firm.

Your Notes...

Simple Sugar Candy Drops

Makes: about 20 candies

Ingredients

- 1 cup sugar.
- ⅓ cup water.
- 1 tablespoon honey.

Instructions

1. Place the sugar, water, and honey in a small saucepan.
2. Heat over medium heat, stirring until the sugar has completely dissolved.
3. Once dissolved, allow the mixture to come to a gentle boil. Stop stirring and let it cook until it forms a thick syrup and turns a light golden colour. This usually takes about 5–8 minutes.
4. Line a tray with baking paper.
5. Carefully spoon small drops of the hot syrup onto the baking paper, leaving space between each drop.
6. Allow the candy to cool and harden completely at room temperature.
7. Once set, peel the candy drops from the baking paper.

Hard Caramel Lollies

Serves: 12

Ingredients

- 1 cup sugar.
- ¼ cup water.

Method

1. Place the sugar and water in a small saucepan.
2. Heat over medium heat, stirring until the sugar dissolves.
3. Allow the mixture to simmer without stirring until it turns a deep golden caramel colour.
4. Carefully spoon small circles onto baking paper or pour into lightly greased candy moulds.
5. Allow the lollies to cool and harden completely.

Storage

Store in an airtight container in a cool, dry place.

Your Notes...

Caramel Using Sweetened Condensed Milk

This simple caramel is made using sweetened condensed milk and can be used as a topping or filling for desserts.

Serves: 6

Ingredients

- 1 can (395 g) sweetened condensed milk.

Method

1. Remove the label from the unopened can of sweetened condensed milk.
2. Place the can in a saucepan and cover completely with water.
3. Bring the water to a gentle boil, then reduce to a simmer.
4. Simmer for **2–3 hours**, ensuring the can remains fully covered with water at all times.
5. Carefully remove the can from the water and allow it to **cool completely** before opening.
6. Once opened, the milk will have thickened into a smooth caramel.

Sauces from Pantry Ingredients

A well-stocked pantry can transform the simplest ingredients into something satisfying. When fresh produce is limited, sauces become the quiet heroes of the kitchen. With a few tins, jars, spices, and staples tucked away in the cupboard, it is possible to create rich tomato bases, smoky barbecue glazes, or tangy, sweet and sour sauces that bring life to pasta, rice, beans, or whatever happens to be on hand.

Pantry sauces are not only practical, but they are forgiving. They invite improvisation, encouraging cooks to adjust sweetness, acidity, or spice according to taste and what is available. The recipes below rely mostly on non-perishable ingredients and simple techniques, making them ideal for quick meals, emergency cooking, or stretching basic staples into something comforting and flavourful.

Your Notes...

Sweet and Sour Pantry Sauce

Ingredients

- ½ cup canned pineapple juice or syrup from canned pineapple
- ¼ cup vinegar (white or apple cider)
- 3 tbsp brown sugar
- 2 tbsp tomato sauce
- 1 tbsp soy sauce
- 1 tbsp cornstarch mixed with 2 tbsp water

Instructions

1. Combine pineapple juice, vinegar, sugar, ketchup, and soy sauce in a saucepan.
2. Bring to a gentle simmer over medium heat.
3. Stir in the cornstarch mixture and cook until thickened.

Use for: stir-fries, meatballs, chicken, or vegetables over rice.

Your Notes...

Honey Garlic Pantry Sauce

Ingredients

- ¼ cup honey
- 3 tbsp soy sauce
- 1 tsp garlic powder
- 1 tbsp vinegar or lemon juice (bottled works)
- 1 tsp cornstarch mixed with 2 tbsp water

Instructions

1. Combine honey, soy sauce, garlic powder, and vinegar in a small saucepan.
2. Simmer for 3–4 minutes.
3. Add the cornstarch mixture and cook until slightly thick.

Use for: chicken, tofu, roasted vegetables, or noodles.

Your Notes...

Simple Teriyaki Sauce

Ingredients

- ¼ cup soy sauce
- 2 tbsp brown sugar
- 1 tbsp honey or sugar
- 1 tsp garlic powder
- ½ tsp ground ginger
- 1 tsp cornstarch mixed with 2 tbsp water

Instructions

1. Combine soy sauce, sugar, honey, garlic powder, and ginger in a saucepan.
2. Simmer for a few minutes.
3. Add cornstarch mixture and cook until glossy and thick.

Use for: stir-fries, rice bowls, or marinades.

Your Notes...

Creamy Pantry Alfredo-Style Sauce

(Made without fresh cream)

Ingredients

- 1 tbsp of oil
- 1 tbsp flour
- 1 cup shelf-stable milk or powdered milk prepared according to directions
- 1/4 cup grated shelf-stable parmesan (or powdered parmesan)
- 1/2 tsp garlic powder
- Salt and pepper

Instructions

1. Melt butter and stir in flour to make a paste.
2. Slowly whisk in milk until smooth.
3. Add parmesan, garlic powder, salt, and pepper.
4. Cook until thick and creamy.

Use for: pasta, baked vegetables, or casseroles.

Your Notes...

Pantry Tomato Sauce

Ingredients (all pantry-friendly):

- 1 can crushed or diced tomatoes (400 g / 14 oz)
- 1 tbsp olive oil (or any cooking oil)
- 1 tsp garlic powder (or ½ tsp dried minced garlic)
- 1 tsp onion powder
- 1 tsp dried oregano
- ½ tsp dried basil (optional)
- ½ tsp sugar (balances acidity)
- Salt and pepper to taste

Instructions

1. Heat the oil in a saucepan over medium heat.
2. Add garlic powder and onion powder and stir for about **30 seconds**.
3. Add the canned tomatoes.
4. Stir in oregano, basil, sugar, salt, and pepper.
5. Simmer **10–15 minutes**, stirring occasionally until slightly thickened.

Good for: pasta, pizza base, meatballs, or dipping sauce.

Pantry BBQ Sauce

Ingredients

- 1 cup tomato sauce or ketchup
- 2 tbsp brown sugar (or white sugar)
- 1 tbsp vinegar (white or apple cider)
- 1 tbsp soy sauce (adds depth)
- 1 tsp smoked paprika (or regular paprika)
- ½ tsp garlic powder
- ½ tsp onion powder
- ½ tsp black pepper
- Optional: ½ tsp chilli flakes or hot sauce

Instructions

1. Combine all ingredients in a small saucepan.
2. Stir over medium heat until it starts to bubble.
3. Reduce heat and simmer 5–10 minutes until slightly thick.

Good for: grilled meat, baked beans, pulled chicken, burgers, or roasted vegetables.

Flour-Based Survival Meals

Flour is one of the most versatile and reliable staples in a non-perishable pantry. With a few basic ingredients, it can be used to prepare a wide range of simple meals that provide energy and nourishment when fresh foods are limited.

Many flour-based recipes require only a small number of shelf-stable ingredients such as water, oil, powdered milk, or baking powder. These combinations can be used to make breads, flatbreads, dumplings, pancakes, and other filling meals using pantry supplies.

Because flour stores well when kept in airtight containers in a cool, dry place, it is often considered a foundational ingredient in emergency food preparation. Learning a few simple flour-based recipes allows households to create satisfying meals using ingredients that are commonly kept on hand.

Your Notes...

Simple Flour Dumplings

Ingredients

- 1 cup flour
- ½ tsp salt
- ½ cup water

Instructions

1. Mix into a thick dough.
2. Drop spoonfuls into boiling broth or soup.
3. Cook 10 minutes until firm.

Your Notes...

Golden Syrup Dumplings

Ingredients

1. For the dumplings
2. 1 cup self-raising flour
3. Pinch salt
4. 1 tbsp vegetable oil
5. About ½ cup of water
6. For the syrup
7. 1 cup water
8. ½ cup golden syrup
9. ¼ cup brown sugar
10. 1 tbsp butter *(optional)*
11. ½ tsp vanilla *(optional)*

Method

1. Mix flour and salt. Add oil and enough water to form a soft dough. Roll into small balls.
2. In a saucepan, add water, golden syrup, sugar, and butter. Bring to a gentle boil.
3. Drop the dumplings into the boiling syrup.
4. Cover and cook on low heat for 10–12 minutes, until dumplings are soft and cooked through.
5. Stir in vanilla if using and spoon the syrup over the dumplings.

Flour Tortillas

Ingredients

- 1 cup flour
- 1 tbsp oil
- ⅓ cup water
- Pinch salt

Instructions

1. Mix into soft dough.
2. Divide and roll thin.
3. Cook in a hot pan until bubbles form and golden, then flip and cook the other side.

Your Notes...

Basic Pancakes

Ingredients

- 1 cup flour
- 1 tbsp sugar
- 1 tsp baking powder
- ¾ cup water or powdered milk mixture

Instructions

1. Mix ingredients into batter.
2. Cook small portions on a hot skillet.

Your Notes...

Simple Gravy and Bread

Ingredients

- 2 tbsp flour
- 2 tbsp oil or fat
- 1 cup water or broth
- Salt and pepper

Instructions

1. Cook flour and fat until lightly browned.
2. Slowly add water while stirring.
3. Simmer until thick.

Your Notes...

Fry Bread

Ingredients

- 1 cup flour
- ½ tsp baking powder
- ¼ tsp salt
- ½ cup water

Instructions

1. Mix the dough and flatten.
2. Fry in oil until golden.

Your Notes..

Survival Noodles

Ingredients

- 1 cup flour
- 1 egg equivalent in egg powder(or extra water if unavailable)
- Pinch salt

Instructions

1. Mix the dough and roll it thin.
2. Cut into strips.
3. Boil 3–4 minutes in salted water or soup.

Your Notes...

Thickening Roux

Ingredients

- 2 tbsp flour
- 2 tbsp oil or butter

Instructions

1. Cook flour and fat together until golden.
2. Add to soups or stews to thicken.

Simple Drop Biscuits

Ingredients

- 1 cup flour
- 1 tsp baking powder
- ½ tsp salt
- ½ cup water or milk

Instructions

1. Mix into thick dough.
2. Drop spoonfuls onto baking pan.
3. Bake 12–15 minutes at 400°F (200°C).

Skillet Cornbread (Flour Version)

Ingredients

- 1 cup flour
- 1 tbsp sugar
- 1 tsp baking powder
- ¾ cup milk or water

Instructions

1. Mix ingredients.
2. Pour into a greased skillet.
3. Bake or cook covered on the stovetop until firm.

Simple Pasta Dough

Ingredients

- 1 cup flour
- 1 egg, egg powder or ½ cup water
- Pinch salt

Instructions

1. Knead dough until smooth.
2. Roll thin and cut shapes.
3. Boil until tender.

Quick Survival Pizza Base

Ingredients

- 1 cup flour
- 1 tsp baking powder
- ½ cup water
- 1 tbsp oil

Instructions

1. Mix the dough and press it into skillet.
2. Add canned toppings if available.
3. Cook covered until the crust firms.

Simple Crackers

Ingredients

- 1 cup flour
- ¼ cup water
- 1 tbsp oil
- Pinch salt

Instructions

1. Roll the dough very thin.
2. Cut squares.
3. Bake at 170 °C for 12–15 minutes until crisp.

Your Notes...

Onion or Vegetable Fritters

Ingredients

- 1 cup flour
- ¾ cup water
- Salt and spices
- Chopped onions or canned vegetables

Instructions

1. Mix batter and vegetables.
2. Fry spoonfuls in oil until golden.

Your Notes...

Simple Sweet Dough

Ingredients

- 1 cup flour
- 2 tbsp sugar
- 1 tbsp oil
- ½ cup water

Instructions

1. Mix the dough and form small rounds.
2. Bake or pan-cook until golden.

Your Notes...

Campfire Stick Bread

Ingredients

- 1 cup flour
- ½ cup water
- Pinch salt

Instructions

1. Roll dough into strips.
2. Wrap around a stick.
3. Cook over fire until browned.

Your Notes...

Flour and Egg Scramble

Ingredients

- 2 tbsp flour
- 4 tbsp egg powder mixed with
- Salt and pepper

Instructions

1. Mix eggs and flour.
2. Cook in a skillet like scrambled eggs.

Thick Survival Soup Base

Ingredients

- 3 tbsp flour
- 3 cups water or broth
- Salt and spices
- Any canned vegetables or meat

Instructions

1. Whisk flour with a small amount of water.
2. Add remaining liquid and ingredients.
3. Simmer until thick and hearty.

Meals You Can Make in Under 20 Minutes

A well-stocked pantry allows you to prepare quick and satisfying meals with minimal effort. Many shelf-stable foods cook quickly or are ready to eat, making them ideal for busy days or situations when fresh ingredients are unavailable.

The following meal ideas use common non-perishable foods such as canned vegetables, beans, pasta, rice, and shelf-stable proteins. Most of these meals require only basic cooking equipment and can be prepared in about 20 minutes or less.

Tuna and Crackers Plate

Ingredients

- Canned tuna
- Crackers
- Optional: mustard, mayonnaise packets, or hot sauce

Instructions

Drain the tuna and mix with seasoning or condiments if available. Serve with crackers for a quick and protein-rich meal.

Your Notes.....

Rice and Beans Bowl

Ingredients

- Cooked rice
- Canned black beans or kidney beans
- Salsa or canned tomatoes
- Spices such as cumin or chilli powder

Instructions

Heat the beans and mix with cooked rice. Add salsa or spices for flavour.

Your Notes....

Peanut Butter Oatmeal

Ingredients

- Instant or rolled oats
- Powdered milk or water
- Peanut butter
- Honey or dried fruit

Instructions

Cook oats with water or powdered milk. Stir in peanut butter and sweeten with honey or dried fruit.

Your Notes....

Chickpea Salad

Ingredients

- Canned chickpeas
- Olive oil
- Vinegar
- Salt, pepper, or dried herbs

Instructions

Drain and rinse chickpeas. Mix with oil, vinegar, and seasonings for a quick protein-rich salad.

Your Notes...

Lentil Soup

Ingredients

- Dried lentils
- Canned tomatoes
- Canned vegetables
- Spices

Instructions

Simmer lentils in water for about 15 minutes. Add canned vegetables and tomatoes for flavour.

Your Notes...

Ramen Noodle Stir Bowl

Ingredients

- Ramen noodles
- Canned vegetables
- Soy sauce or hot sauce
- Optional canned chicken

Instructions

Cook noodles according to package instructions. Stir in vegetables and protein.

Your Notes....

Rice and Canned Chicken

Ingredients

- Cooked rice
- Canned chicken
- Canned vegetables
- Seasonings

Instructions

Heat chicken and vegetables, then serve over rice.

Your Notes...

Tomato and Bean Soup

Ingredients

- Canned tomatoes
- Canned beans
- Garlic powder or herbs
- Water or broth

Instructions

Combine all ingredients in a pot and simmer for 10–15 minutes.

Your Notes....

Crackers with Nut Butter and Fruit

Ingredients

- Crackers
- Peanut butter or almond butter
- Dried fruit

Instructions

Spread nut butter on crackers and top with dried fruit.

Your Notes...

Pasta with Tuna

Ingredients

- Cooked pasta
- Canned tuna
- Olive oil
- Salt, pepper, or herbs

Instructions

Mix cooked pasta with tuna and olive oil. Add seasoning to taste.

Your Notes...

Vegetable Rice Bowl

Ingredients

- Cooked rice
- Canned mixed vegetables
- Soy sauce or seasoning

Instructions

Heat vegetables and serve over rice with sauce.

Your Notes...

Split Pea Soup

Ingredients

- Dried split peas
- Canned vegetables
- Seasonings

Instructions

Cook split peas in water until soft, about 15–20 minutes. Add vegetables and spices, and cook for another 10 minutes, stirring.

Your Notes...

Quick Bean Wrap Filling

Ingredients

- Canned refried beans or mashed beans
- Salsa
- Seasonings

Instructions

Heat beans and mix with salsa. Serve with crackers or flatbread if available.

Your Notes....

Pantry Trail Mix Bowl

Ingredients

- Nuts
- Dried fruit
- Granola or cereal

Preparation

Mix ingredients for a quick snack or light meal.

Your Notes...

Emergency Pantry Meals for Pets

During emergencies, disasters, or unexpected shortages, pet food may not always be available. Having a basic understanding of how to prepare temporary meals for pets using pantry staples can help ensure that dogs and cats continue to receive nourishment until regular food supplies are restored.

These recipes are **not intended for long-term feeding**, but they can safely sustain pets for short periods when commercial pet food is unavailable.

Important Safety Notes

Before preparing food for pets, remember a few key guidelines:

- **Avoid toxic foods.** Never feed pets onions, garlic, chocolate, grapes, raisins, alcohol, or foods containing xylitol.
- Keep **seasoning** minimal. Pets do not need salt, spices, or sauces.
- Introduce changes slowly if possible to prevent stomach upset.
- Provide fresh water at all times.

Dogs are omnivores and can tolerate a wider variety of foods than cats. Cats are obligate carnivores and require higher levels of protein.

Planning ahead for Pets

When building an emergency pantry, remember that pets rely entirely on their owners for food and water. Including them in preparedness planning ensures they remain healthy and comfortable during uncertain times.

Even a small reserve of shelf-stable ingredients can help keep **tails wagging and whiskers twitching** until normal routines return.

Emergency Dog Food Recipes

Dogs can safely digest many common pantry foods, which makes it possible to prepare simple meals or treats for them using ingredients that are already stored in the home. Foods such as plain rice, oats, canned meats, and certain vegetables can provide useful sources of carbohydrates, protein, and fibre for dogs when prepared without added seasonings or harmful ingredients.

Grains like rice and oats are often gentle on a dog's digestive system and can be helpful when preparing simple meals, especially if a dog has an upset stomach. These ingredients provide energy and are commonly used in homemade dog foods and treats. Oats also contain fibre, which can help support healthy digestion.

Canned meats such as chicken, tuna, salmon, or other plain preserved meats can provide protein and flavour that many dogs enjoy. These meats should ideally be packed in water rather than oil or heavy sauces, and they should be served without added salt, spices, onions, or garlic, which can be harmful to dogs.

Some vegetables that are commonly found in the pantry, including canned carrots, green beans, peas, or pumpkin, can also be used in small amounts to add nutrients and fibre. When using canned vegetables, it is best to choose varieties without added salt whenever possible and to rinse them if they contain excess sodium.

While many pantry foods can be safely shared with dogs, it is important to avoid ingredients that are known to be toxic to them. Foods such as chocolate, onions, garlic, grapes, raisins, and artificial sweeteners like xylitol should never be given to dogs.

By using simple pantry staples and avoiding harmful ingredients, it is possible to prepare basic meals or treats for dogs when commercial pet food or treats may not be available. These options can be especially useful during emergencies or situations when regular supplies are temporarily limited.

Your Notes...

Simple Rice and Meat Meal

Ingredients

- 1 cup cooked rice
- ½ cup canned chicken, tuna, or salmon (packed in water)
- ¼ cup canned vegetables such as carrots, peas, or green beans

Instructions

1. Cook rice according to package directions.
2. Drain canned meat.
3. Mix rice, meat, and vegetables together.
4. Allow the mixture to cool before serving.

This simple meal provides carbohydrates, protein, and fibre.

Your Notes...

Oatmeal and Peanut Butter Energy Meal

Ingredients

- 1 cup cooked plain oatmeal
- 1 tablespoon natural peanut butter (xylitol-free)
- ¼ cup canned pumpkin or mashed sweet potato

Instructions

1. Prepare plain oatmeal with water.
2. Stir in peanut butter and pumpkin.
3. Allow to cool before feeding.

Pumpkin supports digestion, and peanut butter provides healthy fats.

Your Notes...

Pantry Stew for Dogs

Ingredients

- 1 cup cooked pasta or rice
- ½ cup canned beans (well rinsed)
- ½ cup canned chicken, tuna, or sardines
- ¼ cup canned vegetables

Instructions

1. Combine all ingredients in a bowl.
2. Mash lightly so the mixture is easy to eat.
3. Serve once cooled.

Your Notes...

Peanut Butter Oat Dog Biscuits

Ingredients

1 cup rolled oats

1 cup flour

½ cup peanut butter (unsweetened, no xylitol)

½ cup water

2 tbsp powdered milk (optional)

Instructions

1. Preheat oven to **180°C / 350°F**.
2. Mix all ingredients in a bowl until dough forms.
3. Roll the dough and cut into small shapes.
4. Place on a baking tray.
5. Bake for **20 minutes** until firm.
6. Allow to cool before serving.

Your Notes...

Tuna Pantry Dog Treats

Ingredients

1 can of tuna in water (drained)

1 cup flour

½ cup oats

¼ cup water

Instructions

1. Preheat oven to **180°C / 350°F**.
2. Mash tuna in a bowl.
3. Mix in flour, oats, and water.
4. Roll into small balls or flatten into biscuit shapes.
5. Bake for **15–20 minutes**.

Your Notes...

Sardine Dog Biscuits

Ingredients

1 can of sardines in water

1 cup flour

½ cup oats

¼ cup powdered milk (optional) or water

Instructions

1. Mash sardines well.
2. Mix in flour, oats, and powdered milk.
3. Add a small amount of water if needed to form dough.
4. Shape into small biscuits.
5. Bake **20 minutes at 180°C / 350°F**.

Your Notes...

Simple Cornmeal Dog Biscuits

Ingredients

1 cup cornmeal

1 cup flour

½ cup powdered milk (optional) replace with water

½ cup water

Instructions

1. Mix ingredients together to form dough.
2. Roll out and cut into shapes.
3. Bake **20–25 minutes at 180°C / 350°F**.

Your Notes...

Quick Survival Dog Treat

Ingredients

½ cup peanut butter

½ cup oats

¼ cup powdered milk

Instructions

1. Mix ingredients until thick.
2. Roll into small balls.
3. Serve as small treats.

Important Safety Note for Dogs

Avoid using the following ingredients in dog treats:

- Chocolate
- Onions or garlic
- Grapes or raisins
- Artificial sweeteners such as **xylitol**

Always ensure peanut butter **does not contain xylitol**, which is toxic to dogs.

Your Notes...

Emergency Cat Food Recipes

Cats have different nutritional needs from dogs and require a diet that is much higher in protein. As natural carnivores, cats depend primarily on meat or fish to provide the nutrients their bodies need to stay healthy. For this reason, meals prepared for cats should focus mainly on animal-based proteins rather than grains or vegetables.

Shelf-stable pantry foods such as canned fish, canned chicken, canned salmon, or other preserved meats can be useful sources of protein for cats when fresh food or commercial pet food is not available. These foods should ideally be packed in water rather than oil or heavy sauces and served plain without added seasonings. Cats are particularly sensitive to ingredients such as onions, garlic, and certain spices, which should always be avoided.

While small amounts of grains such as rice may occasionally be used to stretch a meal if supplies are limited, they should only make up a very small portion of a cat's diet. Cats rely heavily on animal protein to obtain essential nutrients such as taurine, which supports healthy heart function, vision, and overall wellbeing.

Some canned fish varieties, such as tuna or sardines, can be used as occasional meals or treats for cats, but they should not be the sole food source for long periods. Whenever possible, a variety of protein sources should be offered to help maintain a more balanced diet.

In emergency situations where commercial pet food may be unavailable, simple meals made from plain canned meats or fish can help ensure that cats continue to receive the protein they require. Providing fresh drinking water alongside these foods is also important to support proper hydration.

By keeping a few suitable protein-rich pantry items on hand, households can help ensure that their cats remain fed and cared for even when regular pet food supplies may be temporarily disrupted.

Your Notes...

Sardine and Rice Mash

Ingredients

- ½ tin sardines in water (not oil)
- 1–2 tablespoons cooked rice
- 1 tablespoon canned pumpkin (optional)

Instructions

1. Drain the sardines and mash them with a fork.
2. Mix with cooked rice and pumpkin.
3. Serve in small portions.

Sardines are rich in protein and healthy fats that help support a cat's energy levels.

Your Notes...

Salmon and Oatmeal Mix

Ingredients

- ½ can salmon (packed in water)
- 1 tablespoon cooked plain oatmeal

Instructions

1. Drain the salmon and remove any large bones.
2. Flake the fish into small pieces. Mix with cooked oatmeal.
3. Allow to cool before serving.

This recipe provides protein with a small amount of carbohydrates for additional energy.

Your Notes...

Simple Chicken and Rice Meal

Ingredients

- ½ cup canned chicken
- 1 tablespoon cooked rice
- 1 tablespoon canned carrots (mashed)

Instructions

1. Shred the chicken into small pieces.
2. Mash the carrots thoroughly.
3. Mix all ingredients together and serve.

Your Notes....

Chicken and Lentil Protein Bowl

Ingredients

- ½ cup canned chicken
- 1 tablespoon cooked lentils
- 1 tablespoon mashed pumpkin or sweet potato

Instructions

1. Shred the canned chicken finely.
2. Mix with well-cooked lentils and pumpkin.
3. Serve at room temperature.

Lentils add fibre and additional nutrients when used in small amounts.

Your Notes....

Simple Fish Meal

Ingredients

- ½ can tuna or salmon (packed in water)
- 1–2 tablespoons cooked rice or oats

Instructions

1. Drain fish.
2. Serve in small portions.

Your Notes....

Chicken Pantry Mix

Ingredients

- ½ cup canned chicken
- 1 tablespoon cooked rice
- 1 tablespoon mashed pumpkin

Instructions

1. Finely shred the chicken.
2. Mix with rice and pumpkin.
3. Serve slightly warm or at room temperature.

Your Notes...

Alternative Cooking Methods

Preparing Meals When the Power Is Out

Most of the time, we rely on modern appliances such as electric stoves, ovens, and microwaves to prepare our meals. However, there may be times when these conveniences are unavailable. Power outages, storms, natural disasters, camping trips, or travel can leave us without access to a traditional kitchen.

Knowing a few alternative cooking methods can make a significant difference during these situations. With a little creativity and some simple equipment, it is still possible to prepare warm and satisfying meals using pantry ingredients.

This chapter explores several practical cooking methods that do not rely on electricity. These techniques have been used for generations in outdoor settings and emergency situations. Many require only simple tools and a safe outdoor space.

Whether you are camping, preparing for emergencies, or simply interested in traditional cooking methods, these approaches can help you continue preparing meals when standard kitchen appliances are not available.

Campfire Cooking

Campfire cooking is one of the oldest and most reliable ways to prepare food. With a safe fire pit and a few simple tools, a wide variety of meals can be prepared outdoors.

Equipment

- Cast iron pot or pan
- Grill grate
- Foil
- Long-handled utensils

Direct Flame Cooking

Food is placed directly over the fire on a grill grate or in a pan.

Good for:

Flatbreads, Damper, Pancakes and Fry bread

Foil Packet Cooking

Ingredients are wrapped in foil and placed in hot coals.

Good for:

Rice meals, Bean dishes and Vegetables

Pot Cooking Over the Fire

A pot is suspended over the fire or placed on a grill grate.

Good for:

Soups, Stews, Curries and Pasta

Safety Tips

- Always cook in a designated fire pit.
- Keep water nearby in case of sparks.
- Never leave a fire unattended.

BBQ or Grill Cooking

A barbecue grill is another excellent alternative cooking method. Even a small charcoal grill can be used to prepare many of the recipes in this book.

Grill Cooking

Food is cooked directly over the heat.

Good for:

Flatbreads, Damper and Skillet meals

Indirect Cooking

Food is cooked next to the heat rather than directly above it.

Good for:

Baking bread, cooking casseroles and Slow-cooking stews

Helpful Equipment

- Cast iron pan
- Dutch oven
- Grill basket

Many dishes normally prepared on a stove can easily be adapted to a grill using a sturdy pan or pot.

Candle Cooking

Candle cooking can provide a small but useful heat source during emergencies. While it will not produce the same heat as a stove, it can warm small portions of food or heat liquids.

Suitable Foods

- Soup, Instant noodles, Oatmeal, Rice pouches, Canned meals

Simple Method

1. Place a candle under a small metal stand or rack.
2. Set a metal cup or small pot above the flame.
3. Heat food slowly while stirring.

Safety Tips

- Always place candles on a stable, heat-resistant surface.

- Never leave candles unattended.
- Keep away from flammable materials.

Solar Cooking

A basic solar cooker can be made using a few simple household materials. This type of cooker works by capturing and concentrating the sun's heat inside a covered container, allowing food to cook slowly using solar energy.

Materials needed:

- A sturdy cardboard box
- Aluminium foil
- Plastic wrap or a clear glass lid
- A dark-coloured cooking pot or pan

How it works:

The inside of the cardboard box is lined with aluminium foil, which reflects sunlight into the box. The pot of food is placed inside, and the top is covered with plastic wrap or glass to create a sealed space that traps the heat. The dark pot absorbs the sunlight and converts it into heat, gradually warming and cooking the food.

When placed in direct sunlight, the cooker acts like a small greenhouse, allowing temperatures to rise enough to slowly cook foods such as rice, beans, soups, or stews.

Solar cooking takes longer than traditional methods, but it requires no fuel and is an excellent option for camping, emergencies, or situations where electricity or gas is not available.

Foods That Work Well

- Rice
- Beans
- Stews
- Lentils
- Baked dishes

Solar cooking is slow but very energy-efficient.

Thermal Cooking (Heat Retention Cooking)

Thermal cooking is a simple and fuel-saving method that uses stored heat to continue cooking food after it has been brought to a boil. Instead of keeping food on the stove for a long time, the heat already in the pot is trapped and retained in an insulated space. This allows the food to continue cooking slowly without using additional fuel or electricity.

This method has been used for generations and is sometimes called "haybox cooking", because in the past, people insulated their pots in boxes filled with hay or blankets to keep the heat in.

Thermal cooking works especially well for foods that normally simmer for a long time, such as rice, beans, lentils, soups, stews, and grains.

Method

1. Place the food and liquid in a pot and bring it to a full rolling boil on a stove or other heat source.
2. Allow the food to boil for several minutes so it is thoroughly heated.
3. Remove the pot from the heat and secure the lid tightly to keep the heat inside.
4. Wrap the pot in thick towels, blankets, or insulation, or place it inside an insulated container such as a cooler or thermal cooker.
5. Leave the pot undisturbed for several hours while the trapped heat slowly continues cooking the food.

During this time, the pot retains its heat, allowing the food to soften and cook through without additional energy. Thermal cooking is particularly useful during power outages, camping trips, or emergencies, because it greatly reduces the amount of fuel needed for cooking while still producing warm, satisfying meals.

This method is excellent for Rice, Lentils, Soups, Stews

It saves fuel and works well during power outages.

Your Notes...

Portable Gas Stoves

Small camping stoves are one of the easiest emergency cooking options.

Advantages

- Quick and reliable heat
- Easy to control temperature
- Compact and portable

Good Uses

- Boiling water
- Cooking rice or pasta
- Making soups and curries
- Frying bread or pancakes

Cleaning and Hygiene from Pantry and Laundry Staples

When preparing for emergencies, people often focus on food and water. While these are essential, maintaining cleanliness and sanitation is just as important.

During disasters, illness is often caused by poor hygiene, contaminated surfaces, and unwashed hands rather than lack of food alone. If supply chains are disrupted or stores are closed, everyday cleaning products may become difficult to obtain. Simple items such as dish soap, laundry detergent, or hand soap can quickly become essential household supplies.

Fortunately, many homes already contain the ingredients needed to maintain cleanliness and hygiene. Long before modern commercial cleaning products existed, households relied on simple, durable ingredients to clean their homes and clothing. Many of these ingredients are still commonly found in laundry rooms and kitchen cupboards today.

Items such as washing soda, borax, baking soda, soap flakes, vinegar, and salt are inexpensive, widely available, and have an extremely long shelf life. In fact, most of them can be stored for years without losing effectiveness. These simple compounds can perform dozens of cleaning tasks, from washing dishes and clothing to scrubbing surfaces and eliminating odours.

In an emergency situation, these humble staples become extremely valuable. With only a few ingredients, it is possible to make:

- All-purpose cleaners
- Dishwashing powders
- Laundry detergent
- Hand soap
- Degreasers
- Scrubbing pastes
- Odour removers
- Stain treatments

These homemade cleaners are not only practical during emergencies; they are also similar to the cleaning methods used by earlier generations. For decades, households maintained clean kitchens, fresh laundry, and sanitary homes using simple mixtures made from mineral powders, soap, and water.

Another advantage of these ingredients is their versatility. A single box of washing soda or borax can serve multiple purposes throughout the home. This makes them ideal for preparedness storage, where space and efficiency matter. Instead of storing dozens of specialised cleaning products, a few core ingredients can perform many different tasks.

Keeping your environment clean during difficult times helps prevent illness, protects food supplies from contamination, and improves morale. When people are forced to live in close quarters or deal with limited resources, maintaining basic sanitation becomes one of the most important ways to safeguard health.

The recipes and methods in this section show how simple pantry and laundry staples can be transformed into effective cleaning and hygiene products. These mixtures require minimal ingredients and equipment, making them practical even when modern conveniences are limited.

By learning how to use these long-lasting ingredients, you can ensure that your household remains clean, healthy, and functional—even when the unexpected occurs.

All-Purpose Cleaner

Basic vinegar cleaner

Mix:

- 1 cup white vinegar
- 1 cup water

Uses:

- Kitchen counters
- Glass
- Bathroom surfaces
- Removing odours

Extra-strength scrub

Mix:

- ½ cup baking soda
- 2 tbsp salt
- Enough vinegar to make a paste

Uses:

- Sinks
- Cookware
- Stubborn stains

Natural Disinfecting Spray

While not as strong as commercial disinfectants, acidic solutions help reduce bacteria.

Mix:

- 1 cup white vinegar
- 1 tbsp lemon juice
- 1 cup water

Store in a spray bottle if available.

Good for:

- Bathroom surfaces
- Cutting boards
- Door handles

Dishwashing Paste

If dish soap runs out, a simple abrasive cleaner can still remove grease and food.

Mix:

- ½ cup baking soda
- 1 tbsp salt
- A small amount of water or vinegar to form a paste

Use with a cloth or sponge.

Laundry Emergency Cleaner

Clothing can be cleaned even without detergent.

Option 1: Baking soda soak . Add:

- ½ cup of baking soda to a bucket of water

Soak clothes for 30 minutes, then rinse.

Option 2: Vinegar rinse. Add:

- ½ cup vinegar to rinse water

Helps remove odour and residue.

Toothpaste Substitute

When toothpaste runs out:

Mix:

- 2 tbsp baking soda
- Pinch of salt
- A few drops of water

Optional:

- drop of peppermint extract if available

Use a small amount on a toothbrush.

Your Notes...

Deodorant Alternative

Baking soda body deodoriser

- Lightly apply baking soda to underarms.

Or, Mix:

- 2 tbsp baking soda
- 1 tbsp cornstarch

Helps absorb moisture and odour.

Dry Shampoo

Useful when water is limited.

Use:

- Cornstarch or baking soda

Method:

1. Sprinkle a small amount onto the scalp.
2. Massage into roots.
3. Brush out excess powder.

Hand Cleaning When Soap is Limited

Sugar or salt scrub

Mix:

- 1 tbsp sugar or salt
- a small amount of cooking oil

Removes grease and dirt effectively.

Odour Control for Rooms

Place small bowls of:

- Baking soda
- Coffee grounds
- Dry tea leaves

These absorb unpleasant smells.

Your Notes...

Emergency Surface Scrub

For tough grime:

Mix:

- Baking soda
- salt
- a small amount of vinegar

Creates a foaming abrasive cleaner.

Your Notes...

Water Storage and Purification

Water is one of the most important supplies to prepare for emergencies. While food can often be stretched or substituted, the human body can only survive a short time without safe drinking water. Disruptions to water supply can occur during natural disasters, infrastructure failures, or other emergencies.

For this reason, it is important to store an adequate supply of clean water and to understand simple ways to treat or filter water if needed.

How Much Water to Store

A common recommendation is to store at least four litres of water per person per day. This amount covers drinking, basic food preparation, and minimal hygiene.

For emergency planning, households may consider storing:

- 3 days of water for short-term disruptions.
- 1–2 weeks of water for extended emergencies.

Remember to include water for pets and household animals when calculating storage needs.

Water Storage Options

Clean water can be stored in a variety of containers. Suitable options include:

- Food-grade water storage containers.
- Large sealed water jugs.
- Bottled drinking water.
- Clean, sealed containers designed for long-term storage.

Store water in a cool, dark location away from direct sunlight and chemicals. Containers should be tightly sealed and clearly labelled.

Rotating Stored Water

Stored water should be checked and rotated periodically to maintain freshness. Many households choose to rotate water every 6–12 months.

When rotating stored water:

- Empty and clean containers if necessary.
- Refill with fresh drinking water.
- Label containers with the storage date.

Water Filtration and Purification

In some situations, stored water may run out or additional water sources may be required. Several methods can help make water safer to drink.

Boiling

Boiling water for **at least one minute** helps kill many harmful microorganisms.

Water Filters

Portable water filters can remove sediment, bacteria, and some contaminants. These filters are commonly used for camping or emergency preparedness.

Water Purification Tablets

Chemical purification tablets or drops can disinfect water when boiling is not possible.

Household Filtration Systems

Some households choose to keep gravity-fed filters or countertop filtration systems for emergency use.

Additional Water Preparation Tips

- Keep a small supply of bottled water that can be used immediately.
- Store extra water for cooking and hygiene.
- Keep portable containers that can be used to collect water if needed.
- Include water storage in your overall emergency preparedness plan.

Planning for water needs helps ensure that households remain safe and prepared during unexpected disruptions.

Y

Comprehensive Non-Perishable Pantry Storage Guide

Protein Sources		
Item	**Storage Method**	**Shelf Life**
Canned tuna	Cool, dry pantry	3–5 years
Canned salmon	Cool, dry pantry	3–5 years
Canned chicken	Cool, dry pantry	3–5 years
Canned sardines	Cool, dry pantry	3–5 years
Canned mackerel	Cool, dry pantry	3–5 years
Canned anchovies	Cool, dry pantry	3–5 years
Canned corned beef or canned beef	Cool, dry pantry	3–5 years
Canned ham	Cool, dry pantry	3–5 years
Spam or luncheon meat	Cool, dry pantry	3–5 years
Canned turkey	Cool, dry pantry	3–5 years
Canned roast beef	Cool, dry pantry	3–5 years

Canned ham chunks	Cool, dry pantry	3–5 years
Canned sausage	Cool, dry pantry	3–5 years
Canned Sausage	Cool, dry pantry	3–5 years
Shelf-stable bacon	Cool, dry pantry	5–10 years
Freeze-dried chicken	Sealed cans or Mylar bags	25–30 years
Freeze-dried beef	Sealed cans or Mylar bags	25–30 years
Canned beans (black beans, kidney beans, chickpeas)	Pantry shelf in original cans	3–5 years
Baked beans	Pantry shelf in original cans	3–5 years
Refried beans	Pantry shelf in original cans	3–5 years
Dried beans (kidney, black, pinto, navy)	Airtight container or Mylar bags	10–30 years
Lentils	Airtight container	10–20 years
Red lentils	Airtight container	8–10 years
Green lentils	Airtight container	10–20 years

Dried peas (split or whole)	Airtight container	10–20 years
Soybeans or dried soybeans	Airtight container	10–15 years
Peanut butter or other nut butters	Cool, dry pantry	1–2 years
Nuts (almonds, peanuts, walnuts, cashews)	Airtight container in cool storage	6–12 months
Seeds (sunflower, pumpkin, chia)	Airtight container	1–2 years
Sesame seeds	Airtight container	1–2 years
Flaxseeds	Airtight container	6–12 months
Textured vegetable protein (TVP)	Airtight container	10–20 years
Shelf-stable tofu	Cool, dry pantry	6–12 months
Chickpea flour (gram flour)	Airtight container	1–2 years
Beef jerky or biltong	Sealed packaging	1–2 years
Dried sausage or salami	Cool, dry pantry	6–12 months

Dried fish or salted cod	Airtight container	1–2 years
Dried shrimp	Airtight container	1–2 years
Fish flakes or powdered fish	Airtight container	2–5 years
Powdered eggs	Sealed container or Mylar bags	5–10 years
Freeze-dried scrambled egg s	Cool, dry pantry. Sealed cans	
Powdered milk	Airtight container or Mylar bags, Cool, dry pantry	10–20 years
Shelf-stable protein bars	Original packaging Cool, dry pantry	6–12 months
Powdered peanut bu tter	Airtight container Cool, dry pantry	5–10 years

Carbohydrates		
Item	**Storage Method**	**Shelf Life**
Rice	Airtight container or Mylar bags	4–5 years
Instant rice	Pantry shelf	5–10 years

Brown rice	Airtight container	6–12 months
Wild rice	Airtight container	10+ years
Pasta or noodles	Airtight container	8–15 years
Egg noodles	Pantry shelf	5–8 years
Ramen or instant noodles	Pantry shelf	1–2 years
Rolled oats or instant oats	Airtight container	10–20 years
Steel-cut oats	Airtight container	10–20 years
Quinoa	Airtight container	5–10 years
Barley	Airtight container	8–10 years
Bulgur wheat	Airtight container	8–10 years
Couscous	Airtight container	5–8 years
Farro	Airtight container	6–10 years
Freekeh	Airtight container	6–10 years
Polenta	Airtight container	5–10 years
Cornmeal	Airtight container	1–2 years

Grits	Airtight container	1–2 years
Flour or baking mix	Airtight container	1 year
Pancake mix	Airtight container	1–2 years
Biscuit mix	Airtight container	1–2 years
Self-raising flour	Airtight container	6–12 months
Breakfast cereal	Sealed packaging	6–12 months
Granola	Airtight container	6 months
Crackers or rice cakes	Sealed packaging	6–12 months
Crispbread	Sealed packaging	8–12 months
Pretzels	Sealed packaging	6–12 months
Breadsticks	Sealed packaging	6–12 months
Shelf-stable tortillas or flatbreads	Pantry shelf	6–12 months
Shelf-stable pita bread	Pantry shelf	6–12 months
Breadcrumbs	Airtight container	1–2 years

Stuffing mix	Airtight container	1–2 years
Instant mashed potatoes or potato flakes	Sealed packaging	10–15 years
Dehydrated potato slices	Mylar bags or an airtight container	15–20 years
Wheat berries	Mylar bags with ox ygen absorbers	30+ years
Whole wheat flour	Airtight container	1 year
Spelt grain	Airtight container	10+ years
Sorghum grain	Airtight container	10–15 years
Millet	Airtight container	10+ years
Amaranth	Airtight container	10+ years
Instant polenta	Airtight container	5–8 years
Hardtack or survival biscuits	Airtight container	20+ years

Vegetables		
Item	**Storage Method**	**Shelf Life**

Canned vegetables (corn, peas, green beans)	Cool, dry pantry	3–5 years
Canned carrots	Cool, dry pantry	3–5 years
Canned potatoes	Cool, dry pantry	3–5 years
Canned mushrooms	Cool, dry pantry	3–5 years
Canned pumpkin	Cool, dry pantry	3–5 years
Canned mixed vegetables	Cool, dry pantry	3–5 years
Canned beets	Cool, dry pantry	3–5 years
Canned spinach	Cool, dry pantry	2–3 years
Canned tomatoes (whole, diced, crushed)	Cool, dry pantry	18–24 months
Tomato paste	Cool, dry pantry	2–3 years
Tomato sauce	Cool, dry pantry	2–3 years
Passata or crushed tomatoes	Cool, dry pantry	18–24 months
Sun-dried tomatoes	Airtight container	1–2 years

Jarred roasted peppers	Cool, dry pantry	1–2 years
Jarred olives	Cool, dry pantry	1–2 years
Pickles or gherkins	Cool, dry pantry	1–2 years
Sauerkraut	Cool, dry pantry	1–2 years
Freeze-dried vegetables	Mylar bags or sealed cans	20–30 years
Dehydrated onions	Airtight container	10–15 years
Dehydrated garlic	Airtight container	10–15 years
Dehydrated carrots	Airtight container	10–15 years
Dehydrated cabbage	Airtight container	10–15 years
Freeze-dried corn	Sealed cans or My lar bags	25–30 years
Freeze-dried peas	Sealed cans or My lar bags	25–30 years

Fruit		
Item	**Storage Method**	**Shelf Life**
Canned cherries	Cool, dry pantry	2–3 years

Fruit cocktail	Cool, dry pantry	2–3 years
Fruit cups or fruit in juice	Cool, dry pantry	1–2 years
Applesauce	Cool, dry pantry	1–2 years
Fruit spreads or jam	Cool, dry pantry	1–2 years
Marmalade	Cool, dry pantry	1–2 years
Dried fruit (raisins, apricots, cranberries)	Airtight container	1–2 years
Sultanas	Airtight container	1–2 years
Currants	Airtight container	1–2 years
Dried apples	Airtight container	1–2 years
Dried bananas	Airtight container	1 year
Banana chips	Airtight container	6–12 months
Dried mango	Airtight container	1–2 years
Dried pineapple	Airtight container	1–2 years
Dates	Airtight container	1–2 years
Prunes	Airtight container	1–2 years

Freeze-dried fruits	Mylar bags or sealed cans	20–30 years
Fruit leather	Airtight container	1 year
Freeze-dried strawberries	Sealed cans or Mylar bags	25–30 years
Freeze-dried blueberries	Sealed cans or Mylar bags	25–30 years
Freeze-dried apples	Sealed cans or Mylar bags	25–30 years

Dairy and Dairy Alternatives		
Item	**Storage Method**	**Shelf Life**
Powdered milk	Airtight container or Mylar bags	10–20 years
Powdered cheese or cheese sauce	Airtight container	5–10 years
Evaporated milk	Cool, dry pantry	1–2 years
Sweetened condensed milk	Cool, dry pantry	1–2 years
UHT milk (long-life milk)	Cool, dry pantry	6–12 months
Shelf-stable cream or cooking cream	Cool, dry pantry	6–12 months
Jarred cheese spread	Cool, dry pantry	1–2 years
Processed shelf-stable cheese	Cool, dry pantry	1–2 years
Shelf-stable butter powder	Airtight container	5–10 years
Ghee (clarified butter)	Cool, dark pantry	1–2 years
Shelf-stable margarine or spreads	Cool, dry pantry	6–12 months

Coconut milk (canned)	Cool, dry pantry	2–5 years
Coconut cream	Cool, dry pantry	2–5 years
Powdered coconut milk	Airtight container	5–10 years
Shelf-stable almond milk	Cool, dry pantry	6–12 months
Shelf-stable soy milk	Cool, dry pantry	6–12 months
Shelf-stable oat milk	Cool, dry pantry	6–12 months
Shelf-stable rice milk	Cool, dry pantry	6–12 months

Fats and Cooking Oils		
Item	**Storage Method**	**Shelf Life**
Cooking oil (vegetable, canola, sunflower)	Cool, dark place	1–2 years
Olive oil	Cool, dark place	18–24 months
Coconut oil	Cool, dark place	2–5 years

Avocado oil	Cool, dark place	1–2 years
Sesame oil	Cool, dark place	1 year
Shortening	Sealed container	2–3 years
Lard or cooking fat	Cool storage	1–2 years
Butter powder	Airtight container	5–10 years
Nut and seed butters	Cool, dry pantry	1–2 years
Shelf-stable butter (canned butter)	Airtight container	10 years
Powdered shortening	Cool pantry	10+ years

Condiments and Flavourings		
Item	**Storage Method**	**Shelf Life**
Salt	Airtight container	Indefinite
Sugar	Airtight container	Indefinite
Honey	Sealed jar	Indefinite
Maple syrup	Cool, dry pantry	1–2 years
Molasses	Cool, dry pantry	2–5 years

Vinegar (white, apple cider, malt)	Cool, dry pantry	Indefinite
Balsamic vinegar	Cool, dry pantry	Indefinite
Soy sauce or tamari	Cool, dry pantry	3–5 years
Worcestershire sauce	Cool, dry pantry	3–5 years
Mustard (powdered or jarred)	Cool, dry pantry	1–2 years
Ketchup	Cool, dry pantry	1 year
BBQ sauce	Cool, dry pantry	1 year
Hot sauce or chilli sauce	Cool, dry pantry	3–5 years
Chilli oil	Cool, dark pantry	1–2 years
Salsa	Cool, dry pantry	1 year
Jarred pasta sauce	Cool, dry pantry	1–2 years
Curry paste or curry sauce	Cool, dry pantry	1–2 years
Stir-fry sauce	Cool, dry pantry	1–2 years
Bouillon cubes or broth powder	Airtight container	2–5 years

Soup base or paste concentrate	Cool, dry pantry	1–2 years
Instant soup packets	Cool, dry pantry	1–2 years
Dried herbs and spices	Airtight container	2–4 years
Garlic powder	Airtight container	3–4 years
Onion powder	Airtight container	3–4 years
Paprika	Airtight container	2–3 years
Cumin	Airtight container	3–4 years
Oregano	Airtight container	2–3 years
Basil	Airtight container	2–3 years
Thyme	Airtight container	2–3 years
Chilli flakes	Airtight container	2–3 years
Black pepper	Airtight container	3–4 years
Cinnamon	Airtight container	3–4 years
Nutmeg	Airtight container	3–4 years
Miso paste	Cool pantry	1–2 years
Fish sauce	Pantry storage	2–3 years

Hoisin sauce	Pantry storage	1–2 years
Teriyaki sauce	Pantry storage	1–2 years
Nutritional yeast	Airtight container	2–3 years

Baking Essentials		
Item	**Storage Method**	**Shelf Life**
Baking powder	Airtight container	1–2 years
Baking soda	Airtight container	Indefinite
Dry yeast	Airtight container	1–2 years
Cornstarch	Airtight container	Indefinite
Brown sugar	Airtight container	Indefinite
White sugar	Airtight container	Indefinite
Powdered sugar	Airtight container	Indefinite
Cocoa powder	Cool, dry pantry	2–3 years
Chocolate chips	Cool, dry pantry	1–2 years

Desiccated coconut or flakes	Airtight container	6–12 months
Vanilla extract	Cool, dry pantry	Indefinite
Almond extract	Cool, dry pantry	Indefinite
Golden syrup	Cool, dry pantry	Indefinite
Honey	Sealed jar	Indefinite
Dried fruit for baking	Airtight container	1–2 years
Nuts for baking	Airtight container	6–12 months
Powdered butter	Airtight container	5–10 years
Powdered shortening	Airtight container	10 years
Cream of tartar	Airtight container	Indefinite
Gelatine powder	Airtight container	3–5 years
Agar Agar (plant-based gelatine)	Airtight container	2–3 years

Ready-made Meals		
Item	**Storage Method**	**Shelf Life**
Canned soups	Cool, dry pantry	3–5 years
Canned stews	Cool, dry pantry	3–5 years
Canned chili	Cool, dry pantry	3–5 years
Shelf-stable meal pouches	Cool, dry pantry	1–3 years
Instant rice or grain pouches	Cool, dry pantry	1–2 years
Instant noodle cups	Cool, dry pantry	1–2 years
Instant pudding mix	Cool, dry pantry	1–2 years
Gelatine dessert mix	Cool, dry pantry	1–2 years
Instant custard powder	Cool, dry pantry	1–2 years
Packet pasta meals	Cool, dry pantry	1–2 years
Packet rice meals	Cool, dry pantry	1–2 years

Freeze-dried full meals	Sealed pouches or cans	25– 30 years
MRE meals (military style)	Cool storage	5– 8 years
Instant soup cups	Pantry storage	1– 2 years
Dehydrated soup mixes	Airtight container	10– 15 years

Snacks and Quick Food		
Item	**Storage Method**	**Shelf Life**
Granola bars or protein bars	Sealed packaging	6–12 months
Crackers	Sealed packaging	6–12 months
Popcorn kernels	Airtight container	2 years
Microwave popcorn	Cool, dry pantry	1 year
Nuts and trail mix	Airtight container	6–12 months
Roasted chickpeas	Airtight container	6–12 months
Dried fruit snacks	Airtight container	1 year
Shelf-stable snack cakes	Cool, dry pantry	6 months
Hard candy	Airtight container	5+ years
Chocolate bars	Cool, dry storage	1–2 years

Beverages		
Item	**Storage Method**	**Shelf Life**
Coffee or instant coffee	Airtight container	10–20 years
Ground coffee	Sealed container	6–12 months
Decaffeinated coffee	Sealed container	6–12 months
Coffee pods (for manual brewers)	Cool, dry pantry	1 year
Instant cappuccino or latte mix	Cool, dry pantry	1–2 years
Chicory coffee or grain coffee substitutes	Airtight container	2–5 years
Tea (black, green, herbal, chai)	Airtight container	2–3 years
Instant iced tea mix	Cool, dry pantry	2–3 years
Cocoa mix or hot chocolate mix	Cool, dry pantry	1–2 years
Cocoa powder	Cool, dry pantry	2–3 years
Drinking chocolate	Cool, dry pantry	1–2 years

Milo or malt chocolate drink powder	Cool, dry pantry	1–2 years
Malted milk drink powder	Cool, dry pantry	1–2 years
Powdered drink mixes or electrolyte drinks	Cool, dry pantry	2–5 years
Sports drink powders	Cool, dry pantry	2–5 years
Vitamin drink mixes	Cool, dry pantry	2–3 years
Energy drink powder sticks	Cool, dry pantry	1–2 years

The Stuff Preppers Brag About		
White rice	Mylar bags with ox ygen absorbers	25–30 years
Hard red wheat berries	Mylar bags with ox ygen absorbers	30+ years
Hard white wheat berri es	Mylar bags with ox ygen absorbers	30+ years
Dried corn	Airtight container or Mylar bags	25–30 years

Rolled oats	Mylar bags with ox ygen absorbers	20–30 years
Steel-cut oats	Mylar bags with ox ygen absorbers	20–30 years
Pinto beans	Mylar bags with ox ygen absorbers	25+ years
Black beans	Mylar bags with ox ygen absorbers	25+ years
Kidney beans	Mylar bags with ox ygen absorbers	25+ years
Lentils	Mylar bags with ox ygen absorbers	25+ years
Split peas	Mylar bags with ox ygen absorbers	25+ year
Chickpeas	Mylar bags with ox ygen absorbers	25+ year
Dehydrated potato flak es	Mylar bags with ox ygen absorbers	20–30 year
Freeze-dried vegetables	Sealed cans or Myl ar bags	25–30 years
Freeze-dried fruit	Sealed cans or Myl ar bags	25–30 years

Freeze-dried chicken	Sealed cans	25–30 years
Freeze-dried beef	Sealed cans	25–30 years
Freeze-dried scrambled eggs	Sealed cans	20–25 years
Powdered milk (non-fat)	Mylar bags with oxygen absorbers	20+ years
Powdered eggs	Airtight container	10–20 years
Textured vegetable protein (TVP)	Airtight container	20 years
Dehydrated carrots	Airtight container	15–20 years
Dehydrated onions	Airtight container	15–20 years
Dehydrated cabbage	Airtight container	15–20 years
Instant mashed potatoes	Mylar bags with oxygen absorbers	20+ years
Bouillon cubes	Airtight container	10+ years
Cornstarch	Airtight container	Indefinite
Salt	Airtight container	Indefinite

Sugar	Airtight container	Indefinite
Honey	Sealed container	Indefinite

Household Essentials Checklist

Cooking and Preparation Supplies	
☐ Aluminium foil	☐ Measuring cups
☐ Baking paper	☐ Measuring spoons
☐ Plastic wrap	☐ Kitchen scale
☐ Zip-seal bags	☐ Mixing bowls
☐ Food storage containers	☐ Whisk
☐ Airtight storage jars or containers	☐ Wooden spoon
	☐ Rubber spatula
☐ Vacuum sealing bags	☐ Chef's knife
☐ Manual can opener	☐ Paring knife
☐ Bottle opener	☐ Cutting board
☐ Jar opener	☐ Ice cube trays
☐ Saucepan	☐ Freezer bags
☐ Frying pan	☐ Dishwashing liquid
☐ Large cooking pot	☐ Dishcloths or sponges
☐ Baking trays	☐ Tea towels
☐ Baking dish	☐ Food storage labels or markers
☐ Colander or strainer	

☐ Ladle ☐ Tongs ☐ Serving spoon	☐ Rubber bands or bag clips ☐ Food thermometer ☐ Kitchen timer
Household Checklist	
☐ All-purpose cleaner	☐ Cleaning cloths or microfiber cloths
☐ Dish soap	☐ Spray bottles
Laundry detergent	☐ Rubber gloves
Bleach	☐ Scrub brushes
☐ White vinegar	☐ Sponges
☐ Baking soda	☐ Scrubbing powder
☐ Washing soda	☐ Borax

Personal Hygiene Supplies	
☐ Bar soap	☐ Cotton balls or pads
☐ Liquid hand soap	☐ Hand sanitiser
☐ Shampoo	☐ Wet wipes or baby wipes
☐ Conditioner	☐ Razors
☐ Toothpaste	☐ Cotton swabs
☐ Toothbrushes (extra	☐ Dental floss
☐ Feminine hygiene products	☐ Deodorant
Laundry Supplies ☐ Laundry detergent	**Waste Management Supplies**

	☐ Garbage bags (heavy-duty)
☐ Stain remover	☐ Kitchen rubbish bags
☐ Washing soda	☐ Disposable gloves
☐ Borax	☐ Paper towels
☐ Clothespins	☐ Twist ties or bag ties

Basic Health and First Aid Supplies ☐ Adhesive bandages	
☐ Gauze pads	☐ Hydrogen peroxide or antiseptic solution
☐ Medical tape	☐ Pain relievers
☐ Antiseptic wipes	☐ Thermometer
☐ Tweezers	☐ Basic first aid manual

Lighting and Household Utility Items ☐ Flashlights	☐ Matches or lighters
☐ Extra batteries	☐ Extension cords
☐ Battery-powered lanterns	☐ Portable phone chargers or power banks
☐ Candles	
Comfort and Daily Living Items ☐ Notebooks	☐ Pens
☐ Batteries	☐ Sewing kit
☐ Duct tape	☐ Playing cards or small games
☐ Extra blankets	

Prepared Household Checklist

Use this checklist to help build a simple preparedness plan for your home. Having basic supplies on hand can help your household stay safe and comfortable during emergencies such as power outages, severe weather, or unexpected disruptions.

Food & Water

☐ At least **3–7 days of non-perishable food** for each household member

☐ Canned vegetables, fruit, beans, and meats

☐ Dry goods such as rice, pasta, oats, lentils, and flour

☐ Cooking basics (salt, sugar, cooking oil, spices)

☐ Ready-to-eat meals or foods that require little preparation

☐ Manual can opener

☐ Clean drinking water (**at least 3 litres per person per day**)

☐ Additional stored drinking water containers

☐ Collapsible water containers

Water Storage and Purification

☐ Water purification tablets

☐ Portable water filter

☐ Household water filter pitcher

☐ Water purification drops or liquid treatment

☐ Food-grade water storage containers

Cooking & Kitchen

☐ Portable camp stove or backup cooking method

☐ Matches or lighter

☐ Basic cookware suitable for emergency cooking

☐ Paper plates or easy-clean dishes if water is limited

☐ Paper towels

Safety & Lighting

☐ Torch or lanterns

☐ Spare batteries

☐ Battery storage container

☐ Battery or crank radio for emergency information

☐ Candles and safe candle holders

☐ Whistle for signalling help

Home Safety and Emergency Tools

☐ Fire extinguisher

☐ Smoke detectors with working batteries

☐ Carbon monoxide detector

☐ Basic tool kit

☐ Multi-tool or pocket knife

☐ Duct tape

☐ Work gloves

☐ Plastic sheeting

☐ Rope or paracord

Emergency Communication

☐ Written emergency contact list

☐ Local emergency numbers

☐ Family emergency communication plan

☐ Phone chargers or portable power banks

☐ Charging cables for devices

☐ Solar charger or emergency charger

Important Documents

☐ Copies of identification documents

☐ Birth certificates

☐ Passports

☐ Insurance policies

☐ Medical records

☐ Prescription lists

☐ Emergency contact list

☐ Home ownership or rental documents

☐ Printed family contact list

☐ Emergency cash in small bills

Sanitation and Waste Supplies

☐ Heavy-duty garbage bags

☐ Household bleach for disinfecting

☐ Disposable cleaning cloths
☐ Bucket with lid (emergency toilet if needed)
☐ Disposable toilet bags or liners
☐ Laundry detergent

Health and First Aid Checklist

Basic First Aid Supplies

☐ Adhesive bandages (various sizes)

☐ Sterile gauze pads

☐ Adhesive medical tape

☐ Elastic bandages (compression bandages)

☐ Antiseptic wipes or solution

☐ Antibacterial ointment or cream

☐ Burn cream or burn gel

☐ Sterile dressings

☐ Cotton balls or cotton pads

☐ Medical gloves (disposable)

☐ Tweezers

☐ Small scissors

☐ Safety pins

☐ Digital thermometer

☐ Instant cold packs

☐ First aid manual or guide

Medicines and Treatments

☐ Pain relief medication (paracetamol or ibuprofen)

☐ Anti-inflammatory medication

☐ Antihistamines for allergies

☐ Cough medicine or cough drops

☐ Cold and flu medication

☐ Decongestants

☐ Anti-diarrhoea medication

☐ Oral rehydration salts or electrolyte powders

☐ Antacid tablets

☐ Motion sickness tablets

☐ Hydrocortisone cream for skin irritation

☐ Calamine lotion for itching or rashes

☐ Personal prescription medications

☐ Spare inhalers if required

Hygiene and Health Supplies

☐ Hand sanitiser

☐ Antibacterial soap

☐ Disinfectant wipes

☐ Tissues

☐ Face masks

☐ Disposable gloves

☐ Feminine hygiene products

☐ Incontinence products if needed

☐ Toothbrushes

☐ Toothpaste

☐ Dental floss

☐ Lip balm

☐ Sunscreen

☐ Insect repellent

Additional Health Supplies

☐ Eye wash or sterile saline solution

☐ Eye drops

☐ Nasal saline spray

☐ Heat packs or heating pads

☐ Reusable ice packs

☐ Medical information list (allergies, medications, conditions)

☐ Emergency contact information

Children and Baby Supplies

☐ Infant formula or toddler milk

☐ Baby food jars or pouches

☐ Baby cereal

☐ Bottles and bottle nipples

☐ Bottle brush and cleaning supplies

☐ Diapers or pull-ups

☐ Baby wipes

☐ Diaper rash cream

☐ Pacifiers or comfort items

☐ Child-safe medications

☐ Favourite toys or comfort items

Elderly or Special Care Needs

☐ Prescription medications

☐ Mobility aids (walking sticks, walkers)

☐ Spare glasses or hearing aid batteries

☐ Incontinence products if needed

Pet Food and Care Supplies

☐ Dry pet food (dogs or cats)

☐ Canned or wet pet food

☐ Pet treats

☐ Long-lasting chew treats or dental chews

☐ Pet food storage containers (airtight)

☐ Portable pet water bottles or bowls

☐ Extra pet food bowls

☐ Pet vitamins or supplements

☐ Pet medications (flea, tick, heartworm treatments)

☐ Pet first aid kit

☐ Pet bandages or gauze

☐ Pet-safe antiseptic solution

☐ Tick remover tool

☐ Pet nail clippers

☐ Pet brush or grooming tools

☐ Pet shampoo or wipes

☐ Extra collars and ID tags

☐ Spare leash or harness

☐ Pet waste bags

☐ Litter and Portable litter tray or extra litter box

☐ Pet bedding or blankets

☐ Pet carrier or crate

☐ Pet comfort items (favourite toys or blankets)

☐ Emergency pet records (vaccination records, microchip number)

☐ Photo of your pet for identification

Emergency Shelter and Warmth

☐ Warm blankets or extra clothing

☐ Rain gear or waterproof jackets

☐ Spare socks and warm layers

☐ Sleeping bags

☐ Emergency thermal blankets

☐ Tarps or waterproof coverings

Comfort and Morale Supplies

☐ Books or reading materials

☐ Playing cards or board games

☐ Notebooks and pens

☐ Small toys for children

☐ Comfort foods or treats

☐ Family photos or sentimental items

References and Resources

The information in this book is based on commonly accepted food safety practices, emergency preparedness guidelines, and traditional cooking methods. Readers wishing to learn more about food storage, nutrition, and emergency preparedness may find the following resources helpful.

Food Standards Australia New Zealand (FSANZ). (2023). *Food Safety Standards and Safe Food Storage.* https://www.foodstandards.gov.au

Australian Government Department of Health and Aged Care. (2023). *Food Safety and Safe Food Handling.* https://www.health.gov.au

Eat For Health – Australian Government National Health and Medical Research Council (NHMRC). (2023). *Australian Dietary Guidelines.* https://www.eatforhealth.gov.au

Safe Food Australia – FSANZ. (2023). *Guide to Food Safety Standards.* https://www.foodstandards.gov.au

Australian Red Cross. (2023). *Emergency RediPlan: Preparing Your Household for Emergencies.* https://www.redcross.org.au

Australian Government – Get Ready Australia. (2023). *Emergency Preparedness and Household Kits.* https://www.getready.gov.au

State Emergency Service (SES). (2023). *Emergency Preparedness and Home Emergency Kits.*
(Example: NSW SES)
https://www.ses.nsw.gov.au

Queensland Government. (2023). *Emergency Kit and Food Supplies.* https://www.qld.gov.au/emergency

U.S. Department of Agriculture (USDA). (2023). *Food Storage Guidelines for Consumers.* https://www.usda.gov

FoodKeeper App – USDA & Cornell University. (2023). *Food Storage Guidance.* https://www.foodkeeper.app

Centers for Disease Control and Prevention (CDC). (2022). *Food and Water Safety During Power Outages.* https://www.cdc.gov

Solar Cookers International. (2023). *Solar Cooking Basics.* https://www.solarcookers.org

Boy Scouts of America. (2016). *Camp Cooking Handbook.*

Edelstein, S. (2015). *Cooking with the Sun: Solar Cooking Basics*. Solar Cookers International.

DeLong, D. (2010). *How to Survive Without a Refrigerator.* Storey Publishing.

Morris, J. (2008). *Basic Country Skills: A Practical Guide to Self-Reliance*. Skyhorse Publishing.

Australian Veterinary Association (AVA). (2023). *Nutrition and Feeding Advice for Dogs and Cats.* https://www.ava.com.au

RSPCA Australia. (2023). *Feeding Your Dog.* https://www.rspca.org.au

RSPCA Australia. (2023). *Feeding Your Cat.* https://www.rspca.org.au

RSPCA Australia. (2023). *Foods that are Dangerous to Pets.* https://www.rspca.org.au

NSW Department of Primary Industries. (2023). *Responsible Pet Ownership and Animal Care.* https://www.dpi.nsw.gov.au

Agriculture Victoria. (2023). *Caring for Dogs and Cats.* https://agriculture.vic.gov.au

Pet Medical Crisis – Animal Poisons Helpline Australia. (2023). *Toxic Foods for Pets.* https://animalpoisons.com.au

Made in the USA
Monee, IL
04 November 2026

67385827R00223